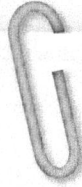

Fit4Work
Fit4Life

by Tina Blake

Fit4Work Fit4Life
Stress free living in the modern world

2nd edition published in 2010 by Tell Me More

Hillditch Cottage, Hillditch Lane, Hartlebury DY11 7YD

www.fit4workfit4life.com

Printed and Bound by Lightning Source in the UK and USA

Photography copyright © Fotolia.com

Set in Helvetica Neue 11pt on 14pt by Charlotte Mouncey

Printed on acid-free paper from managed forests. This book is printed on demand, so no copies will be remaindered or pulped.

ISBN 978-0-9566100-0-3

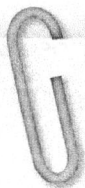

To Debbie Waltier
and her Son

Disclaimer

The author recognises that in the fields of science and medicine there are widely differing opinions. The author believes in a natural and holistic approach to health, energy and vitality. None of the information contained in this book is intended to diagnose, prevent, treat, or cure any disease. Before making any changes in prescribed drugs, diet or exercise it is highly recommended that you consult with your medical practitioner. Whilst all reasonable care has been taken in the preparation of this publication neither the publisher nor the author can accept any responsibility for any loss occasioned to any person acting or refraining from action as a result of relying upon its contents.

Contents

Foreword

I have written this book because I feel passionate about life and I feel passionate about health. I feel passionate about health because for 7 years of my life I had to live without it.

I am not an exercise fanatic and I do not live on lettuce leaves. I am someone who wants to work hard, have a good social life and do my sports. I think I am someone like you. Of course there will be differences, you might not do a sport but still enjoy a walk now and again, even if it's only to pick up a paper. You might find the gym a great place to be, or a necessary evil. You might think that life is a bit of a drag, or that it's one big party, but, basically, what I think we have in common is that we want to enjoy the time we have, in whatever way suits us.

Born on 1st July 2005 I have discovered at least some of the secrets to a happier, healthier existence. That is, of course, not my real birth date, but the date that I emerged from a severe bout of Myalgic Encephalomyelitis (ME), also commonly known as Chronic Fatigue Syndrome (CFS), to re take control of my own life.

I had achieved much in my previous years, working for over 20 of them as a successful corporate communicator. I have worked, and still do work, for some of the top companies in the world. I work as a writer, a video director and as a presentation trainer through my company Tell Me More. (www.tellmemoreltd.co.uk) In much of my work I come into direct contact with the enormous effect that our minds can have over our bodies. I work one on one with many of my clients, helping them to overcome a corporate problem, a personal fear, a perception or an illness and I have seen them benefit from the ideas I offer in this book.

I have learned the hard way that it doesn't matter how successful you are in life, illness can take it all away from you. Without your mental and physical health you have nothing.

Before Myalgic Encephalomyelitis (ME) hit me, I had many, many warning signals that I was abusing both my body and my mind, burning the proverbial candle I guess. I was not necessarily out partying, with wild, late nights and massive hangovers, instead, I was working long hours under pressure, coping with a great deal of emotional upset and not looking carefully enough at what I was eating or at my destructive thought patterns. I firmly believe that I did not need to get as ill as I did. I had the power to prevent it within my own mind and body, I just did not heed the warning signs or apply the knowledge that I had, I convinced myself that stress and illness was something that only other people suffered from.

ME or CFS is widely misunderstood and widely misdiagnosed. It is commonly agreed that it is getting more and more prevalent in the developed world, but does not seem to be on the increase in the third world. This strongly suggests that there is a direct correlation between our modern lifestyle and the onset of this particular body malfunction. I call this malfunction "dis-ease" because very often the dis-ease that your body feels leads to the onset of an actual disease or illness. I believe, and research backs me up, that the chemicals and additives in our over refined food, coupled with our fast paced life style and the quality of the air we breathe all have a contributing factor to our health and well being.

ME is an illness that can strike any person at any time but it tends to afflict people who have undergone a period of high mental or physical stress and it frequently follows a viral infection. Therefore busy people, people who work hard at their careers, people who are go getters and people who neglect their own needs are more likely to suffer. It is more common in women than men and more common in people in their 20s – 40s than in other age groups.

The 'Myalgic' part of the term refers to symptoms associated with muscles. All sufferers endure severe muscle pain and fatigue, an overwhelming sense of tiredness is present more than 20% of the time making it difficult to perform the smallest of tasks. The 'Encephalomyelitis' part refers to brain symptoms which are usually, difficulties with memory, difficulties with concentration and sometimes even difficulties with speech.

I started to feel unwell in 1999 and by 2002 had developed full blown ME. I was virtually bed ridden for 2 years, I was so fatigued that I literally couldn't function. I had a constant sore throat and a feeling of running a temperature, and, although I took my temperature every day for 2 years, it was nearly always normal. I suffered with poor concentration to the point that I could not follow a conversation on the telephone because I had to be able to see the person's facial expressions in order to understand what they were saying. I slept for days at a time, but constantly felt tired and emotional.

I feel passionate about the fact that this did not need to have happened to me. I believe I could have avoided my illness if I had taken better care of myself both mentally and physically. I knew I was run down and yet I did not change one aspect of my lifestyle or one aspect of my thought patterns.

It has taken me several years and much research to make a full recovery and this book is a simple guide to better emotional and physical health. I know that the information will help ME and CFS sufferers, but I have designed it to be much more than that. This life plan can help anyone who suffers the strains of modern life. It can help you if you are basically fit but feel tired and stressed some of the time, and it can help you if you are already debilitated.

I have split the book into 2 sections, the mind and the body, because I know that, just as we are what we eat, we are also what we think. I was, and continue to be, amazed by what I have learnt about the power of the subconscious mind and the influence that you can have over your life just by thinking in the right way. I am also constantly amazed by the massive effect that certain types of food can have on your health, and much more than that, by the fact that the way you eat your food can add vigour to your whole life.

I hope that you enjoy this book and embrace the parts of it that will be of most benefit to you. Every person is different, and every body is different but here I have tried to lay down some general guidelines for a more rewarding life and to enable you to go forward in a way that is beneficial to you and to your overall health.

I wish you every health and happiness.

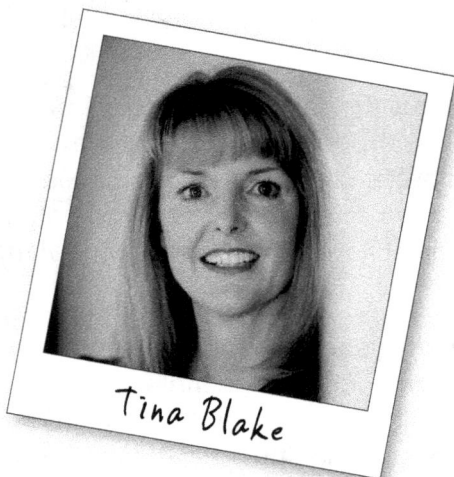

Tina Blake

Icons used in this book

Icons are used throughout this book to bring your attention to important points, facts, tips and questions.

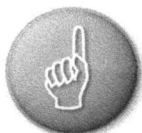

Fact: Knowledge that will help you feel good

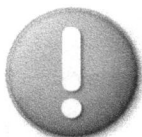

Important: Things you should keep in your mind to help you through each day

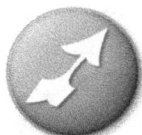

Top tip: A quick fix for some common situations

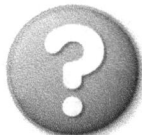

Why?: Common sense answers to frequently asked questions

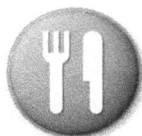

Link: To recipe

The Fit4Work Fit4Life facts

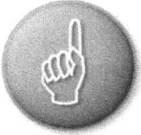

A healthy mind and a healthy body come from within

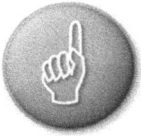

Drugs will only cure a symptom of your problem not the root cause. To cure yourself, you have to look within yourself, look at your lifestyle and look at your mental and physical approach to everything you think and everything you do

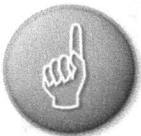

It's not the **size** of the dog in the fight that matters

It's the size of the **fight** in the dog

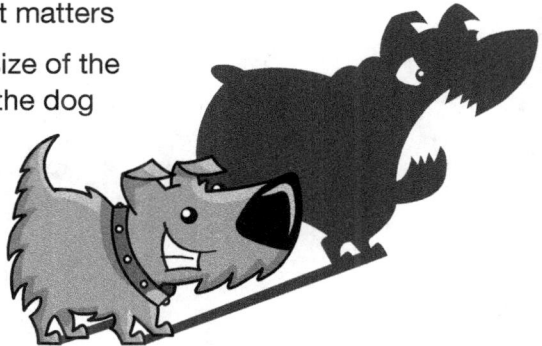

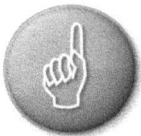

To overcome your anxiety, your lethargy, your stress, all you need is a willingness to learn, to adapt, to change some of your old self and your old lifestyle. Is that too much to ask for a perfect, healthy, vibrant you?

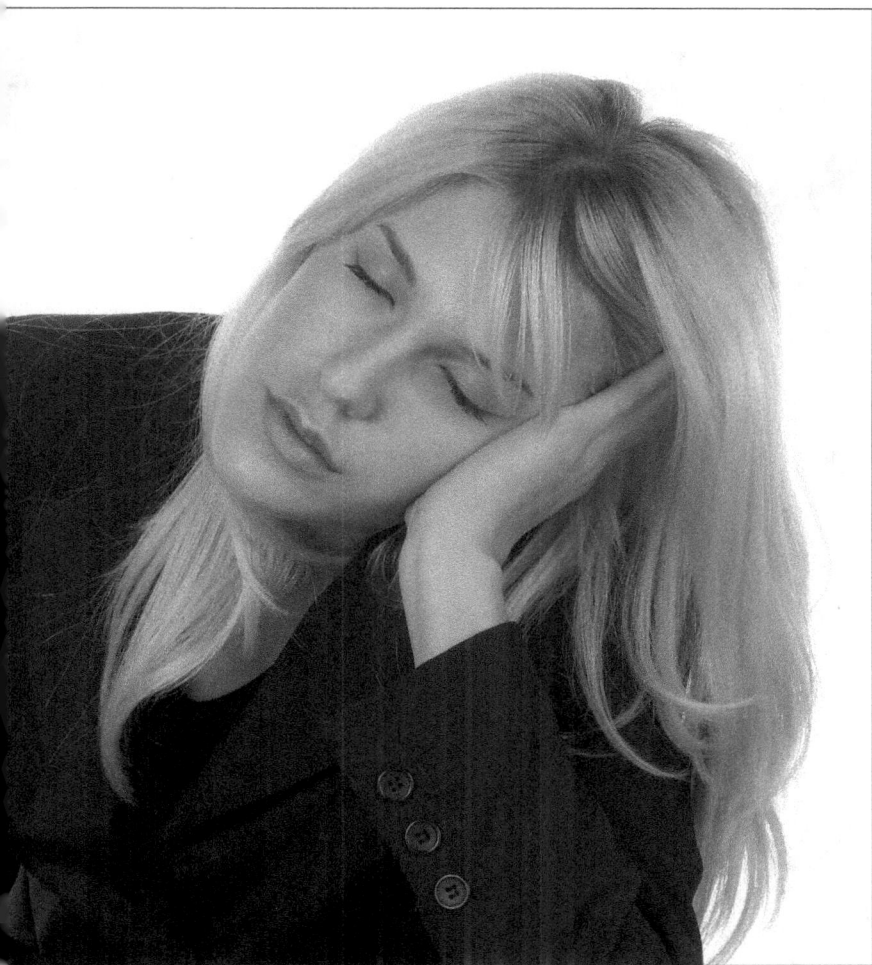

Part I
Every Thought Counts

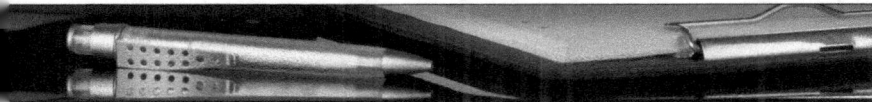

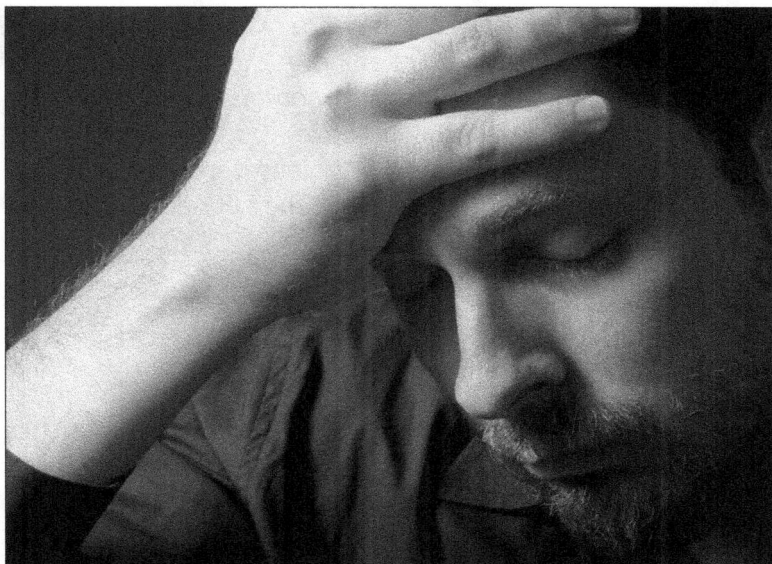

Chapter 1
The overloaded mind and body

An overview of the human predicament

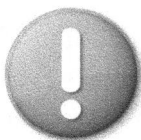

Each year around 175 million working days are lost to illness in Britain alone

In the Swartkrans Cave in South Africa there is evidence that early man was using fire around a million years ago, however it took 850,000 years of evolution to develop man, more or less as we know him, and to find him using fire for cooking and for weapon and pot making. Fast forward again and around 149,000 years later fire was turned into a version of gunpowder by the Chinese to make firecrackers to ward off evil spirits.

By modern day standards man was a pretty slow developer, but the pace of life was quickening. A mere 736 years later Jonathan Hulls patented the Newcomen engine powered, Steam Paddle Boat, sadly it never paddled across the harbour, but 40 years later, engines were installed and working on commercial premises in the UK and Europe and the industrial revolution was underway.

Jump forward 118 years and in 1903 the Wright Brothers took to the air, closely followed, 66 years later by Neil Armstrong walking on the moon.

Technological development may have started slowly, but has accelerated dramatically in the last 50 years and, crucially, our minds and bodies are struggling to keep up with the new demands on them.

Think about the impact that email has had on the average office worker. 50 years ago a request would come in and the respondent had time to read the letter, contemplate the reply, have it typed, think about it again and post it. They would then not expect to hear back from the recipient for at least a day or so. Today a client will ring for a quote or a decision and will expect it by the return press of a button. The pressure on us is immense, and the amount of work and responsibility we are expected to handle in a day has risen dramatically.

The results of this increased pressure are dramatic. Dame Carol Black wrote in her paper Working for a Healthier Tomorrow (2008) that "around 175 million working days were lost to illness in 2006" and that was in Britain alone.

Common sense should tell us that, if we are under constant pressure, we should ensure that we fuel ourselves with the right stuff to handle it. Unfortunately for us, food production has not necessarily improved in the same way that technology has.

1000 years ago, in the UK and Europe, man was actually about as tall as he is now. 9 out of 10 people lived in unpolluted countryside on a simple diet that promoted sturdy limbs healthy teeth and clean lungs. If we jump forward several hundred years to the 16th and 17th Centuries and look at the bones of people who lived then, they show that they were much smaller than we are now. Overcrowding in cities, polluted air and poor food all took a toll on their bodies.

During much of man's evolution he lived mainly off the land, in the countryside. This naturally meant that he ate whatever was in season and so had a constantly varied diet. Refrigeration, as we know it, did not happen until the 1800s and was not in widespread use until the 20th Century. That meant that, for example, man would eat apples and cabbage only when they were in season and fish and animals only when they were passing through his area and have an egg only when his hen laid one. He had a natural selection, and, because of the seasons, his body had a natural rest from certain foods.

By the 17th Century companies like the East India Company were bringing exotic foods from all over the world to Europe. Inter continent trading expanded and in a few short years became the norm. With the advent of refrigeration, it meant that by the 20th Century people could eat apples and cabbage every day of their lives if they wanted to.

The industrial revolution also had a major impact on our food. Man used to grow and thresh his own corn and, naturally, was left with the whole grain. With the advent of flour mills, the grain became more and more refined and, as more people chose to live in the cities, farmers had to produce more food with less labour. Over the next 100 years this led to the introduction of fertilizers to make the land produce more and additives to make the harvested food last longer.

21st Century man now works in an environment polluted by engines, eating over-refined food with many additives and, if he chooses, he can eat the same food every day of his life.

It took 1000s of years for us to develop and learn to cook food, and in just a few hundred we have overloaded our bodies with processed produce and overloaded our minds with the instantaneous demands that technology makes.

The mind and the body are inextricably linked and they are the two most important things we have. Very often we don't believe this until we have abused our bodies so much they show signs of breaking down, or neglected our minds until they become stressed and we lose our sense of calm and well being.

Disease is a warning sign

Many people find that their abuse manifests itself in actual illness or disease, it is your body's way of showing its dis-ease with the pressures upon it. Some of the most common symptoms of dis-ease show as a migraine, sore throat or irritable bowel. Sometimes the abuse manifests itself in imagined or assumed illness. In my case I had the feeling of running a fever for 2 years even though my body temperature was normal.

The physical dis-ease you are feeling when your body has been abused and is out of its natural balance is your body trying to get rid of its toxins, the toxins that you have put into it by your mental and physical lifestyle.

The mental dis-ease that you are feeling when your mind has been abused and is out of its natural balance is your mind warning you that it is overloaded with the wrong type of thoughts.

Main symptoms of dis-ease

The most common bodily symptoms for people suffering from stress at work and a bad diet are:

- *An overwhelming feeling of tiredness, of lethargy*

- *A recurrent sore throat*

- *Muscle aches and pains, especially after physical exertion*

- *Nausea and loss of appetite*

- *Feelings of faintness and dizziness*

The most common mental symptoms of stress at work and bad diet are:

- *A disinterest in work or home life*

- *Feeling depressed*

- *Being unable to control your emotions*

- *Poor concentration*

- *Difficulty in sleeping properly*

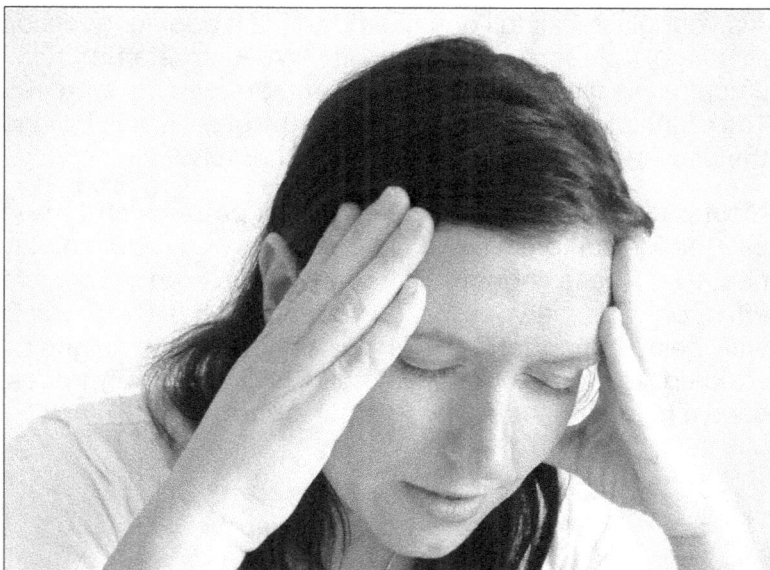

Chapter 2
Your mind

How you affect yourself and others

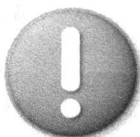

A pessimist is one who makes difficulties of his opportunities
An optimist is one who makes opportunities of his difficulties

Reginald B. Mansell

Your day to day health is governed by both your body and your mind. What you think and how you think it every minute of your life will have a direct effect on your general well being.

"Is your glass half full or half empty?" is a popular question to gauge a person's outlook on life. Whether referring to an actual glass filled with liquid or to a more general concept. The optimist will always answer that the glass is half full and the pessimist will answer that it is half empty.

Most people drop into habitual thought patterns and these can either be predominantly positive, or predominantly negative. These thought patterns will have an immediate effect on your everyday life, on your emotional and physical well being. Importantly, it is not only you that might be affected. How you are thinking and feeling can, and does, have a huge impact on those around you.

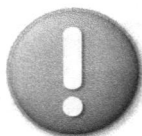

You always take the weather with you

Your "weather" is the way that you communicate with others. It is made up of 2 things, what you actually say or do and the paralanguage that you use when you are saying or doing it. Paralanguage can be the look in your eye, your hand gestures and, most importantly in weather terms, the thought in your head.

We, as humans, believe more of what we see than what we hear so your paralanguage is a really powerful tool. In my corporate training sessions I constantly work with paralanguage and the remarkable effect that it can have on an individual or a group of people.

Think of yourself at work, you are having a bad day, you haven't slept much and your body isn't feeling top form. You have 6 tasks to complete that morning and really you think you only have time for 4 of them, how are you feeling? I would guess anxious, stressed and not at peace with yourself. If a colleague comes over to talk, you are unlikely to look up and give them your best smile and focus all your attention on them, you are quite likely to keep the conversation short, if you have it at all, and to view their visit as an interruption.

Conversely, think of yourself on a day where you haven't slept much and your body isn't feeling top form and you have 6 tasks to complete but think that, actually, you only have time for 4. However, you have just delivered a project which has been well received. You are at your desk feeling pleased with yourself so your other tasks do not seem so imminent. Your colleague comes over to talk. I bet you do give them your best smile and focus on them and tell them about your project and listen to them talk about their work and social life.

It is clear that you will have given off different signals in each scenario - different weather. In the first one, your agitation may well have rubbed off on the colleague who might take it personally and walk away with some of your cloudy, rainy weather in their life through no fault of their own, they could be wondering how they upset you when all they did was stop by to chat. Similarly your sunny good mood could have a great impact on your colleague who, catching your weather, could begin to feel better themselves just for having chatted to you, you could have lifted their mood with your enthusiasm.

Your mental attitude is important to other people, whether you realise it or not, but much more importantly, it is vital to you, and your own well being.

Have you ever noticed that if you are running late for a meeting and you are driving there, every red light seems to be against you and the traffic at every roundabout is blocked up?

Statistically that is not possible – if you completed the same journey when you were not running late, say you had 10 minutes to spare, you wouldn't feel that the whole traffic system was against you in this way, you would not necessarily give the red lights a second thought, you wouldn't notice them because you wouldn't be anxious about being late.

Exactly the same thing is true if your meeting is internal, how many times have you cursed the lift for being slow when you are in a hurry or cursed the person who stops you in the corridor?

What is important to realise is that you give off vibes to other people all the time but most importantly you give off vibes to yourself. The old adage, smile and the world smiles with you is true, but it is even more important that you understand the concept, smile and you smile with yourself.

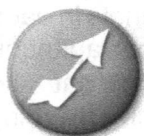

Reduce your stress levels when going to a meeting by allowing extra time for the journey, whether it is up the stairs or 100 miles away.

I know that may not be as easy as it sounds and time management can be a difficult skill to master, but try it and see the difference for yourself.

When I suffered with ME I also suffered with anxiety, the two often seem to be linked, one of my triggers is still being late. I have experimented with this a great deal during my recovery and I know for certain that I am much more able to do a first class job if I arrive in good time with a calm mind and can concentrate on the task in hand. Starting a meeting with an apology is never a good thing.

If you are in the miserable position where you have had to give up work either permanently or temporarily because of your mental and physical condition and find yourself thinking "I wish I could even go to a meeting" don't think that this is not relevant to you. Find something to smile about in your day, and set yourself a task to be done by a certain time, it might be going to get a paper, putting the kettle on or even just going to the bathroom and washing your face. Set yourself a time for the appointment with the shop, kettle or sink and make sure you are punctual, maybe even a little early, it will give you a feeling of achievement.

Your mind can make you sick

The mind is its own place, and in itself
Can make a Heaven of Hell, a Hell of Heaven

John Milton Paradise Lost

You can take control of any situation, you are the only person who is in control of what you think and how you think it. Stress related illness is caused by negative thoughts and negative emotions like anxiety, fear, worry, anger, resentment and jealousy. These emotions wear your body down. They put you in a state of constant alert. When your body is in a state of constant alert it is wearing itself out. These emotions also destroy the balance of your mind. If you are constantly feeling anxiety, fear, worry, anger, resentment or jealousy you are filling your mind with negative thoughts and negative thoughts and emotions become the norm for you. Your mind can easily drop into habitual thought patterns and negativity can become your predominant outlook without you even noticing. You can easily become the pessimist who makes difficulties out of his opportunities. You are what you think, just as you take the weather with you, your emotions can have a massive effect on your health.

Have you ever noticed that you are unlikely to be feeling ill when you are incredibly happy?

How many times are you fine for the "Big Event", whether it is work or pleasure, and then feel washed out and unwell afterwards? That is because your mind is controlling your body, in that case to hold you together when you need it.

This emotional cycle is well documented and many clinical trials have been done to prove it. Some of the most notable are the trials known as the Placebo effect.

Placebo

A placebo is defined as "a substance or procedure a patient accepts as medicine or therapy, but which has no verifiable therapeutic activity."

The word placebo comes from the Latin - I will please. In the 1920's doctors discovered that, in a group of patients who all had the same ailment, and who all believed they could be cured by a particular drug, if half were given the drug clinically known to reduce their symptoms and the other half were given a sugar and water pill -a placebo -there was no significant difference in the recovery rates between the 2 groups. Those who had sugar and water still recovered if they believed they were taking the drug that could help them. The important thing here is the fact that, if they believed they were taking a drug that could help them, they recovered. Their minds were helping their bodies. Positive, happy thoughts aided a recovery.

Nocebo

The nocebo effect is not quite so well documented – nocebo from the Latin - I will harm.

The nocebo effect describes a situation where, in a control group of patients who did not believe in the benefit of the drugs they were taking, a high percentage of those who received the sugar and water pill actually reported that their symptoms had got worse. Without a doubt, your mind can make you sick or your mind can aid your healing process.

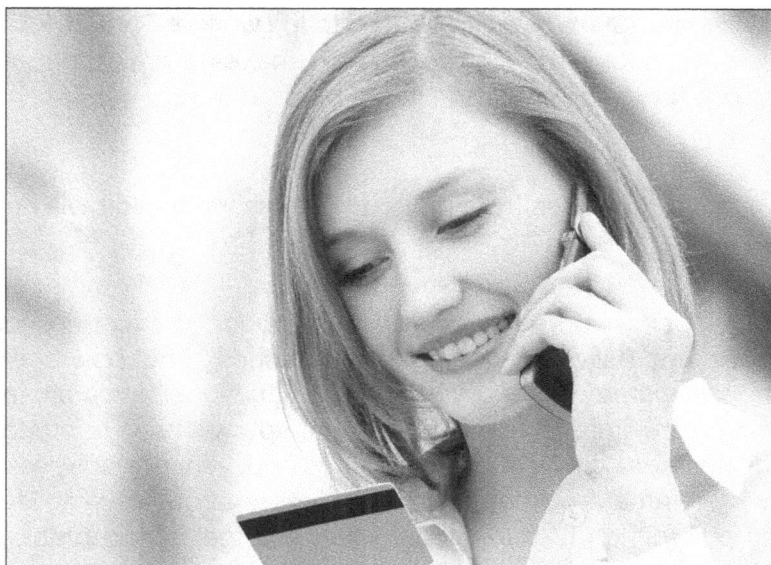

Chapter 3
Living in the Now

There is no past, there is no future - Eckhart Tolle

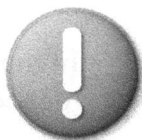

I believe the two most mentally and physically damaging words in the English language are: "WHAT IF...?"

"What if...?" always relates to the past or to the future

"What if...?" is closely linked to negative affirmations: "It's always like that", "it's just the way I am" "whenever I do that xyz happens" "I can't".

In the late 1990's I was introduced to the work of Eckhart Tolle and his book "The Power of Now" makes a great deal of sense for stress free living in the modern world.

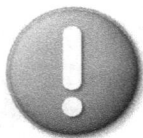

Reality is never as bad as we think it will be

Much of my work involves helping nervous or inexperienced speakers deliver engaging presentations. The power of now is extremely important in these situations. If you are in corporate life it is very possible that you will have to stand up and speak in front of an audience and, very possibly, you will have had, or may still have, doubts about your ability to pull this off to the standard that you feel is acceptable. When I am faced with a client in this situation I work through a series of exercises with them that get them to focus on the now. Invariably they are able to stand up and speak in the now, and from there it is a small step to realise that standing up and speaking the next day, week or month in front of an audience is exactly the same action, it is only their perception of the situation that has changed. Perception is a really important word here and it is totally controlled by your mind. You can be in control of your reaction to any given situation.

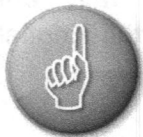

It is not the size of the dog in the fight that matters, it is the size of the fight in the dog

It is how you approach things mentally that will make a massive difference to your success and to your mental and physical well being.

"What if…" will always undermine your mental approach.

How often, when you have been waiting for someone that you love and they are late, have you conjured up their fate? It is a classic "What if...?" scenario.

"What if they have had an accident?"

"What if they are hurt?"

"What if the car has broken down?"

"What if they don't love me and they are not coming?"

The advent of the mobile phone and lap top have made this "What if...?" scenario considerably worse because we expect to be in touch 24/7.

Very often when the person does eventually arrive we are angry with them. That is because we are letting out our emotions, in other words, our thoughts. What we are feeling are the emotions that we ourselves have created. We don't recognise the fact that we have created these thoughts ourselves, and it is these thoughts that have brought us down and made us feel angry, we just let the anger take over. That anger is bringing us further down, both mentally and physically. It is literally wearing us out.

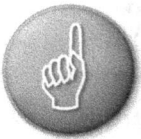

"what if...?" damages your health. When you are thinking about "What if...?" you are not living in the now, you are not appreciating the reality of the situation, you are letting your perception of the situation take over.

Why we should live in the now

If you spend much of your conscious time thinking about the past or the future, invariably your thoughts are not happy ones.

When thinking about the past the thoughts are usually something you perceive that you could have done differently. "What if I hadn't done that", or "What if I had done that". "Whenever I try and do that xyz always happens" If you constantly think about the past you might also dwell upon a time that you perceive to be so good that you would love to be still enjoying it. In both situations perception is key, what you are remembering may not even be what actually happened but what you perceived to have happened and what you are hoping for or dreading may never be going to happen. Both of these thought patterns take you away from reality, from what is actually happening in the now, they take your attention and prevent you from making the most of your current opportunities.

When you are thinking about the future "What if...?" is just as damaging. "What if my idea doesn't work out?" "What if I fail" "what if I can't afford it?" "What if I lose my job?" "What if people laugh at me?" The scenarios are endless but basically a great deal of future thinking involves projecting your fear of the unknown.

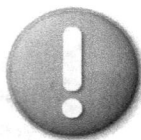

Negative thoughts create fear and fear harms your mind and your mind harms your body. If your thoughts are negative it actually has a real effect on the way you feel, how healthy you feel, how, "up" for the day, you feel. There is a solution – Live in the NOW

Reality is never as bad as we think it is going to be

If you live in the now you also get to fully enjoy some of life's main pleasures, for example joy, happiness, enthusiasm and excitement in the world around you. These emotions are very good for your mind and consequently your body.

They release endorphins which give you a natural high, the same high that you get from doing strenuous exercise.

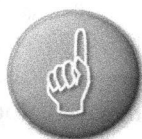

Endorphins are naturally produced bodily chemicals consisting of seretonin and dopemine and basically their effect is to make you feel good.

If you live in the now you are forced to concentrate on what is happening right now, not what made you unhappy a moment before or might cause you a problem a minute or two in the future.

Living in the now takes some practice, at first you have to consciously make yourself do it but the results are worth it.

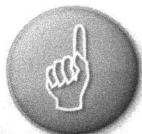

The only place that success comes before work is in the dictionary.

This quote is attributed to several people, which only goes to show how accurate it is. The good news is that to live in the now only takes a small amount of work and the results are phenomenal.

Exercise 1

Whenever you find yourself thinking about something negative – something that has happened or something you fear might happen tell yourself to STOP.

It sounds simple but it is quite difficult to do and will take practice so that you catch your negative thoughts.

Say to yourself STOP and ask yourself if that particular thought is doing you any good at the moment – I can guarantee you that if the thought is negative then the answer is NO!

Then make yourself concentrate on what you are doing in the NOW – it might be driving to your meeting, cleaning your teeth, making a cup of tea, sitting at your desk at work, walking the dog, whatever it is, really think about what you are doing NOW and enjoy it.

If you are out walking really concentrate on the ground under your feet, how does it feel through your shoes? What does the air feel like on your face? How do your clothes feel? What can you see? What can you smell?

The technique works whether you are in a city street, a country park or in your back garden. Make your thoughts go where you want them to go.

With practice many people find it easy to live in the now during the day and then succumb to negative thoughts at the end of the day when they are in bed, tired and off guard. Negative thoughts in bed are just as detrimental to you. Your subconscious mind continues to learn when you are asleep, this is often referred to as subliminal learning. It is very powerful and so you want to make sure that you drift off to sleep dreaming of positive situations and not dwelling on past or future problems.

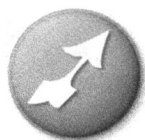

For negative thoughts in bed:

To banish negative thoughts really live in the NOW. Concentrate on the feel of the pillow against your head, and how warm or cool the duvet is. Really think about that and enjoy each sensation. When you feel calm and relaxed deliberately set your mind on a path that you know will aid sleep. This might be thinking about yourself walking along a beach or perhaps drifting in a sailing boat in calm water or visualising something that you particularly enjoy. We will talk more about the power of visualisation and how to achieve it in Chapter 5.

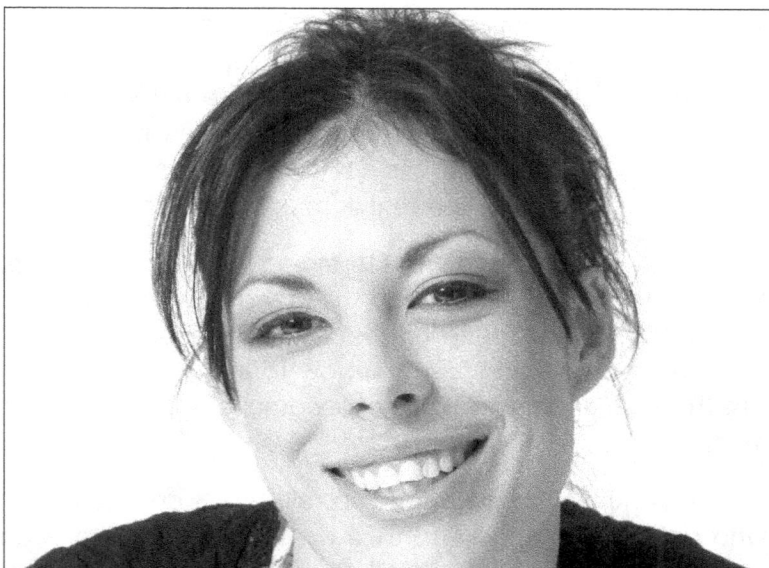

Chapter 4
Think Yourself Well

You are in control

We get what we think we deserve

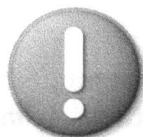

If you think that your life should be good then it will be good. Conversely if you think that your life should be bad, then it will be bad.
We can actually make good or bad happen for ourselves

To recap; much of our stress comes from our PERCEPTION of the situation rather than the situation itself, the, "what ifs…?" that we create around it. For example if you feel stressed about meeting a new boss it is probably because you are "what ifing...?" – what if they don't like me? what if I don't like them? what if they don't like my work? and on and on. The actual meeting, the now as it happens, shaking hands, saying hello is not in itself stressful, it is your perception of the situation that is making you anxious.

You are in control of how much stress there is in your life. You are in control of what you think and how you act. The difficult part is accepting that fact, taking responsibility for your own actions and learning how to influence your own health and happiness, how to become proactive and not reactive.

In the workplace people tend to fall into 2 groups, those who get the job done and those who meet up with each other to discuss how stressed they are. I can guarantee that those in the stress club are sharing their negative thoughts, "I'm so busy, I just can't do it all", "It's gone mad here" "I haven't got enough time to complete that presentation" and of course there will be lots of "What ifing...?" "What if I don't meet the deadline?" "What if I can't get the machine to work?" "What if the computer breaks down?"

Something very similar happens when a group of people with the same illness meet up. Around 80% of them will enjoy swapping stories about their symptoms and difficulties. Their conversation will be predominantly negative, "I can't do that because.." "If I do that I always feel ill"

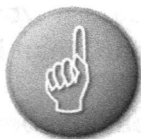

If you constantly think negative thoughts, then your mind will ensure you get what you deserve.

So how does this work?

Your amazing brain

Throughout my working life I have been fascinated with the effect that our minds can have over our bodies, with the way that we communicate both with ourselves and with other people. We can hold ourselves back just by the way we talk to ourselves and conversely we can achieve extraordinary things just by the way we talk, think and approach a subject.

Prior to getting ME I ran my own production company. The nature of that business is that you are constantly pitching for work. I discovered that 90% of the time I won or lost a pitch before I had even walked into the potential client's office to make my presentation.

I discovered that if I genuinely believed I was going to get the business then invariably I would.

This idea is not new and it is not unique to me, it has been around since the days of the bible, but in recent years it has been given an trendy new name, Cosmic Ordering. Cosmic Ordering is based on the Law of Attraction which means that what you put out into the universe you will receive back. The basic principle is that every thought has an energy field which in turn means that we are responsible for creating our world through our beliefs. Literally we get what we think we deserve.

The German author Barbel Mohr made this concept famous in 1995 in her book "The Cosmic Ordering Service" and Noel Edmonds enhanced its fame in the UK when he attributed his success in getting the TV series Deal or No Deal to the power of Cosmic Ordering.

I have tried cosmic ordering myself and have been delighted by the amount of times that it does actually seem to work. My favourite "order" is for a parking space on a busy street.

However, for running my life, personally, I prefer to couple it with a more scientific approach..

When I was bed ridden with ME a friend of mine brought me a book,

"The Power of Your Subconcious Mind" by Joseph Murphy. I had trouble reading and understanding more than a page at a time because of the brain fog associated with my illness, however I grasped the basic message, I could achieve for myself whatever I wanted. All I had to do was to think what I wanted to achieve and really believe that I could achieve it and my subconscious mind would make it happen.

This book put me on the road to getting my health back. It started me on a course of further research to understand how we can take control of our lives.

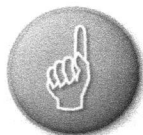

Whatever the mind can conceive and believe, it can achieve.
(Napoleon Hill)

I am not a scientist or a doctor but I had already proved that I could make things happen for myself with my attitude to pitching. It was this belief that I held onto when I was told that I had to accept that I might not walk properly again. It was this belief that led me to discover how "What if…?" can have such a dramatic effect on our mental and physical health.

To explain it, firstly it is necessary to understand a little about how our amazing brain works. I am not an expert on the human brain and, luckily, neither you nor I need to be in order to grasp its basic functioning and to understand why negative thoughts make us ill, why they literally wear us out.

It is widely understood that the brain is split into 2, the conscious mind or thinking brain, and the subconscious mind or reactive brain.

The subconscious mind - approximately 92% of the total brain

Think of the subconscious mind as the vault for your beliefs. It contains your memories, your skills and all your previous life experiences in the limbic or emotional system. In other words anything that is not consciously happening in the now.

It also, according to Paul MacLean's Triune Brain Theory (1953), contains your reptilian brain. Although small, this is a vitally important part of your brain and its interaction with your conscious mind is crucial to your mental and physical health.

No thinking goes on in the reptilian brain, it is purely reactive. It has no desire to do us harm, in fact, its primary function is to keep us alive. It controls the body's autonomic nervous system which means it controls all the things we do automatically like breathing, keeping our hearts beating and digesting food. However, because it does not think for itself, it will produce the reaction that has been requested by the conscious part of our brain without assessing it. This reptilian brain does not learn from its mistakes, if it receives an instruction it will produce the same response again and again.

The Limbic system or emotional brain, sometimes also referred to as the mammal brain, does however learn from its mistakes. It feels and records emotions and creates memories. There is a school of thought that suggests it evolved to help counterbalance the needs of the reptilian brain. For example when the reptilian brain says eat, it will give feelings of pleasure from eating the food thus ensuring that you will do that again. Similarly, because it learns from its mistakes, if you put your hand in fire and burn it your limbic system will remember this and not allow you to do that again.

The concious mind - approximately 8% of your brain

This is also known as the primate brain or neo cortex and frontal lobes This brain controls complex human behaviours like concepts of time, planning, creativity, logic and language. Only human beings have the primate brain, only human beings have the capacity to reason and apply logic in a complex way.

Why we get what we think we deserve

Your conscious mind is the boss in your life and the unconscious mind is the worker that follows orders from it.

We get what we think we deserve because when your conscious mind tells your unconscious mind a negative thing, a "What if...?" then it will act on it without assessing it. Every time you say to yourself or others "What if I can't do it ?", "What if I fail ?" your unconscious mind will receive the negative thought and try to ensure that you get the outcome you have requested, ie failure.

This cycle is extremely damaging to your health and well being. However, this is not the most dangerous aspect of the interaction between the conscious mind and the reptilian part of your unconscious mind.

In the previous chapter we talked about living in the now, about the importance of dealing only with reality in order to maintain mental and physical health. The reasons for this are simple. If your conscious mind is busy with "what ifs...?", conjuring up accidents that may or may not happen and worrying about outcomes of conversations that may or may not take place and dwelling on negative, anxious thoughts, it sends anxious, fearful messages to your unconscious mind, your reptilian brain, and that brain automatically gets your body to react as if there really is a dangerous situation taking place. It does not do it to harm you, it does it automatically, it is a primitive response.

Fight or Flight – a primitive inborn response

Every living creature, whether reptile, mammal or primate is pre programmed with a basic survival instinct which is now known as the fight or flight response. Walter Cannon first described this as the "acute stress response" in the 1920s.

The "fight or flight response" is automatic. It is controlled by the reptilian brain, the non thinking brain, and it is our body's primitive, inborn response that prepares us to "fight" or "flee" from perceived attack. It has been with us since man first evolved, and initially it was the instinct that kept us safe. Through the ages it has helped us survive and feed ourselves. Every animal has it, a deer for example will flee from a lion where as a bear will fight someone or something approaching its cubs. Every animal decides whether to fight or take flight in order to protect itself, and humans are no different.

The Amygdala

The amygdala is part of the unconscious mind, it is located in the mammal, limbic brain, the memory store house. When it receives a message from the reptilian brain that there is danger, it remembers exactly what to do in that situation and releases chemicals like adrenaline, noradrenaline and cortisol into our bloodstream via our nerve cells and our bodies undergo a series of very dramatic changes. We breathe quicker and shallower, blood is directed to our muscles and limbs so that we can either run away or have the strength to fight, our pupils dilate, our sight sharpens and our awareness intensifies so we can scan and search our environment, looking for the enemy.

This is great if we are coping with say a wild bear, or an intruder breaking into our house, but not so great if we are just dealing with our own anxious thoughts.

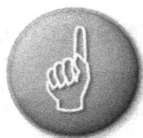

Situations where the amygdala will create adrenaline

PRACTICALLY EVERY SITUATION WHERE YOU ARE NOT LIVING IN THE NOW!

The amygdala will create adrenaline every time you are "what ifing...?" "What if I'm late?", "What if I don't get the contract?", "What if he has had a accident?", "What if I had said something else?", "What if...?", "What if...?", What if...?" you are giving a signal to the reptilian brain that is telling the amygdala that there is danger and that it needs to produce adrenaline to protect you.

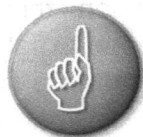

Excess adrenaline causes tiredness, lethargy and feelings of stress

This excess adrenaline, noradrenaline and cortisol is not needed and, because you are not running or fighting, your body can't get rid of it, so it hangs around as a toxic substance in your body. Over time excessive stress toxins lead to disorders of the autonomic nervous system, causing headaches and high blood pressure for example and to disorders of the immune system, the system that protects you from viruses. This makes you more susceptible to catching bugs and can lead to lethargy and, in its developed state, M.E., chronic fatigue, allergies, and even problems like rheumatoid arthritis.

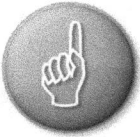

Excess adrenaline causes unwanted bodily reactions

On a moment by moment basis excessive stress toxins also have a huge impact on you. Poor concentration for example is a result of the front of your brain, the conscious mind or primate brain, not getting all the blood flow it needs. It doesn't get the blood flow because it has been sent to your limbs to fight or flee from an imagined danger caused by your anxious thoughts.

The same can happen to your voice, how often have you experienced either yourself or someone else getting a tight or squeaky voice when asked to speak out to a group at work. This is caused because the viscera, (the bit down the middle of your body) has contracted due to lack of blood supply. When they were asked to speak, the person became anxious, the unconscious mind went into fight or flight mode, the amygdala produced adrenaline and the blood flowed away from the viscera and into the limbs.

The unconscious mind thinks it is protecting us but the reptilian brain has not evolved with the pace of modern life, it can now be much more of a hindrance than a help if it is not given the correct signals from our conscious thinking brain.

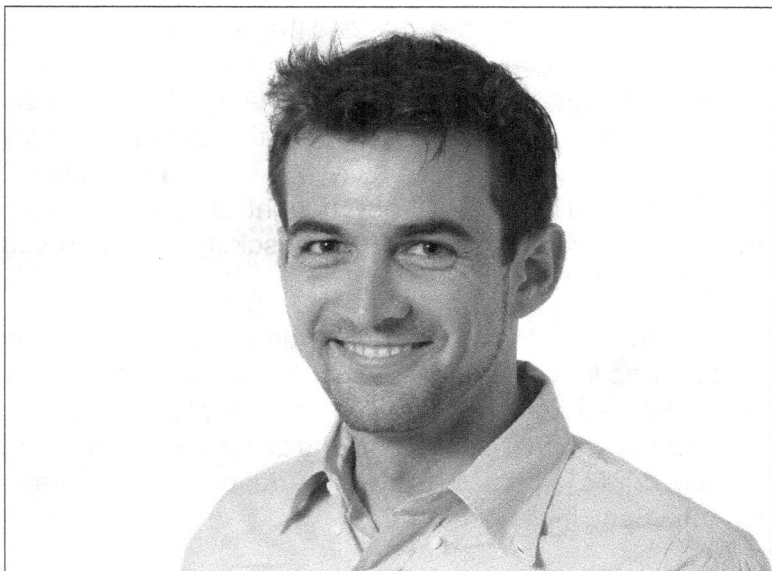

Chapter 5
The Solution

If you keep doing the same thing, you will keep getting the same result

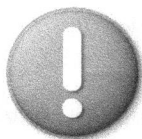

Negative thoughts lead to negative words, which lead to negative actions, which lead to excess adrenaline which leads to a toxic body which leads to stress and lethargy, which in turn leads back to negative thoughts...

To improve our mental and physical health, we need to interrupt this vicious cycle.

In order to bring about the changes that you need you must first make them consciously. To live in the now and outwit the overprotective reptilian brain you need to be consciously aware of when you are thinking negative thoughts. Every time you think something negative you need to stop yourself. If you consciously change your thought pattern it will very quickly have an effect on your unconscious mind and you will get different results.

Each of us has habitual thought patterns, illustrated in broad terms in the glass half full or half empty idea. These habitual thought patterns run along neurological or synaptic pathways between the different parts of our brains. The more habitual our thought patterns are the deeper the grooves or synaptic pathways become.

Reprogramming the synaptic pathways of your brain

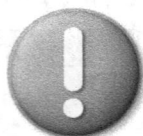

I believe the most important word in any form of self help is CHOICE

Interrupting habitual negative thought patterns by consciously stopping them will interrupt the synaptic pathways. The negative thought will not be able to run all the way to the reptilian brain and cause the usual negative reaction.

Once the thought has been consciously stopped, you have a CHOICE, a very important CHOICE, you can continue with that negative thought and get the negative reaction you always get, or you can replace it with a positive thought.

Replacing negative thoughts with positive ones does not come easily to begin with, you have to make it a habit before it happens subconsciously.

A quick way to discover how negative your habitual thought patterns are is to carry a notebook around with you for a day and write down how you are thinking, how you are talking to yourself. Most people find that their notes are full of "What if...?" and its negative associates: "It's always like that", "it's just the way I am" "whenever I do that xyz happens" and "I can't".

It is important that you write them down as they occur, I think you will be surprised at just how many negative thoughts you have.

When you have your list, take some time to analyse why you have had each negative thought, consciously teach yourself what is going on in your brain.

For example you may have written down "I can't do this" You need to think about **why** you think you can't do it.

Is it because somebody told you that you can't either directly or indirectly?

Is it because you think you have some physical limitation?

Is it because you think you have some mental limitation?

Is it because you are scared?

Is it because you don't want to appear foolish if you fail?

The list of questions is endless, each person is different and each person will have a different reason for thinking negatively about themselves and the situation. There may be deep rooted reasons why you have this particular negative thought, it might have begun in your childhood with your parents, or it might be a relatively new thing in your life, the important thing is to recognise it, and consciously think about it.

Thinking like this on the conscious level will give you an understanding of your self perception and the perception that you bring to each situation that you feel negative about. It will bring results. However, it is not the only tool you have to help you.

Visualisation

Luckily for us, our conscious thoughts, imagination and memory are just as good at creating positive scenarios as negative ones. Creative visualisation is the basic technique underlying positive thinking, it is the technique of using ones thoughts and imagination to visualise specific events that you want to happen, to imagine specific scenarios as you want them to be. I really began to understand the power of visualisation when I ran a series of one on one training sessions with an International sales company doing door to door selling. The people I trained predominantly worked from home and whenever I went to the bathroom in their houses I would find pictures of the life that they wanted to achieve stuck to the back of the toilet door.

I realised that these pictures were a physical embodiment of the mind based scenarios that I had conjured up for myself when pitching for business. I had just seen success, but, by putting these pictures on the backs of their doors, these sales people had a firm idea of what the results of success looked like.

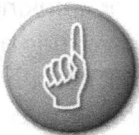

Visualisation allows you to take control of your future. Through visualisation your conscious mind gives your unconscious mind the instructions for what is going to happen. We get what we think we deserve or in other words we tell ourselves what it is we are going to get.

Visualisation is key to a healthy happy life, it works hand in hand with **CHOICE**. You can choose what you want to happen. If you believe in it enough, it will happen for you.

Positive visualisation techniques feature in much of my work. You can apply it to any scenario that you wish. I use it to help people with sporting or corporate challenges and in situations where people have personal and vitality challenges.

You can do the same for yourself. There is a visualisation available as a download on the web site associated with this book. Go to www.fit4workfit4life.com to get your copy. The download will take you through the basic visualisation techniques and give you the tools that you need to become successful in this very powerful technique.

To harness the power of visualisation you first need to be clear about what it is that you want to achieve.

From your list of negative thoughts and your understanding of why you thought like this you should be able to form a clear picture of what it is that you most want, what it is that you feel you could achieve if you were not being held back by feelings of lethargy and stress.

You then need to translate these thoughts into positive images. It may be that you want promotion, it may be a holiday, it may be excellent health, it may be as simple as having enough energy to have friends round for dinner after work in the evening. Really think about where you want your life to take you and then take a pen or pencil or a crayon and draw images representing these things on a piece of paper.

Your drawing technique is not important, stick men and women will do with circles to represent the sun and triangles for the mountains representing a holiday or a few rectangles on top of each other to represent a pile of money, a promotion or a business success. Draw what makes you feel happy.

What you have drawn is the life that is there for you when you follow both parts of this plan, when you take control of your negative thoughts as discussed here in Part I and when you take control of your body in the ways that are discussed in Part II.

What you have drawn are the things that you can make happen for yourself by sending positive messages down your synaptic pathways from your conscious to your unconscious mind. Your unconscious mind will try and fulfill all instructions, without thinking about them, if you have drawn money, then your unconscious mind will try to put you into situations where you will make money.

Do check out the visualisation CD available at www.fit4workfit4life.com which will give you examples of how to use the technique and how to create visualisations that work for you. Remember, the basic principle is to use your imagination to see yourself in a way you would like to be, feeling how you would like to and looking how you would like to.

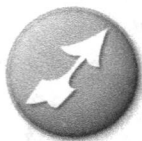

A good time to practice your visualisation is when you are in bed, either before you go to sleep at night or first thing in the morning. Do a "Stop" on your negative thoughts and deliberately set your mind on a path of imagining what you would like to happen. It is best if you actually see yourself in the picture, rather than being an observer, and apply the principles of living in the now – feel the sun on your face if there is sun in your picture and feel the sand between your toes if there is

sand. Hear the sound of the telephone if your picture is in the office and smell the aroma of the food if your picture contains a meal.

When you frequently think of what you would like to happen you are creating a new synaptic pathway, you are making your imagination a reality. Your subconscious mind will make your positive thoughts happen in just the same way as it can bring your negative thoughts to fruition.

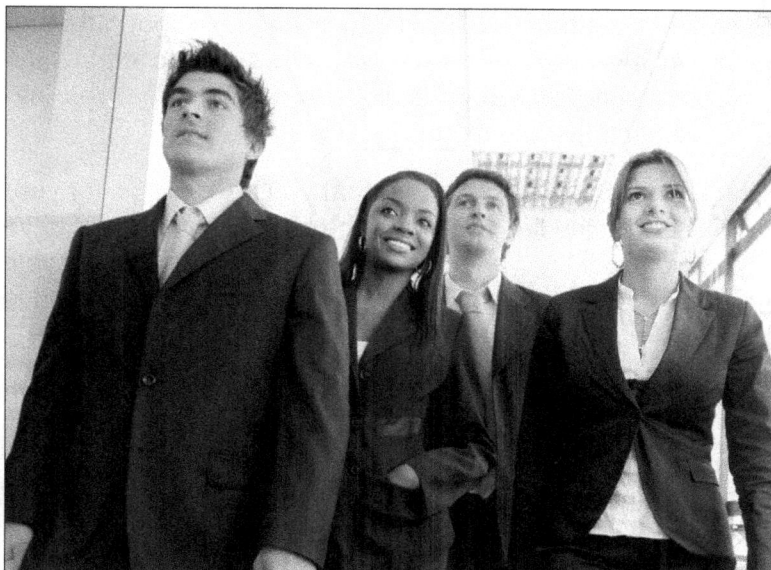

Chapter 6
Creating the Life you Want

A summary of the skills you have learned

How to create the life you want

Exercise 2 in this chapter is a summary of the skills you have learned. It is an exercise that you need to do every time you have a negative thought, it will bring all the elements together and show you that **You** are in control of your life, you can create the life you want.

The exercise builds on exercise 1 and it will be most effective if you have practiced exercise 1 until you have mastered it before you begin exercise 2.

Exercise 1 centered on eradicating negative thoughts and Living in the Now. This exercise allows you to create the outcome that you would like, to turn your negatives into positives and live the life that you will enjoy.

First look at the piece of paper that you have drawn for your visualisation, the life you want, the life that you would have if you were not tired and lethargic, the life you would have if you were not stressed and negative, the life you would have if you were able to.

Study your picture and make sure that you have really drawn the things that you want and take some time to imagine what those things would be like. Really think about the walking or the sunshine or the spending the money, really think about having the energy to do these things and enjoy them.

When you are certain that you have the picture firmly imprinted on your mind use it to help yourself.

Exercise 2

Whenever you find yourself **"what ifing"** thinking about something negative – something that has happened or something you fear might happen tell your mind to **STOP**.

Actually say to yourself the word STOP and think about the now, put yourself in control. I visualise a guillotine coming down and cutting off the negative thought.

In my mind I see the cut end of that negative thought shriveling up, it can no longer go on it's synaptic path.

Now that you are in control, the most important word in any form of self help comes into play, **CHOICE**, you have a **CHOICE**. You can choose to send another negative thought or you can choose to think of something that will help you achieve what you desire, the things that are drawn on the piece of paper

You have the knowledge to understand what is happening to you.

You are in control.

If continue with your negative, fearful thought it will allow your unconscious mind to put you into fight or flight and create adrenaline. It will take blood away from your thinking mind and leave you feeling tired and defeated. Conversely if you consciously direct your thoughts to where you want them to go, you can reinforce your own belief system and see yourself achieving what you want to achieve, your promotion, your holiday, your excellent health.

Taking control of your negative thoughts really is that simple. Interrupt them and replace them and they will lose the physical and mental power that they have over you.

To begin with this will take some conscious effort but as you repeatedly do it your unconscious mind will take over, your unconscious mind will follow instructions from your conscious mind and in a short time it will do much of the work for you. I notice now that every time I start to think something negative, about what I need to achieve, my STOP cuts across automatically. Yes, I still have to think the positive thought because what I want to achieve changes with each success, but ending the negative thought happens before I have consciously thought about it.

It's not the size of the dog in the fight that matters, it's the size of the fight in the dog

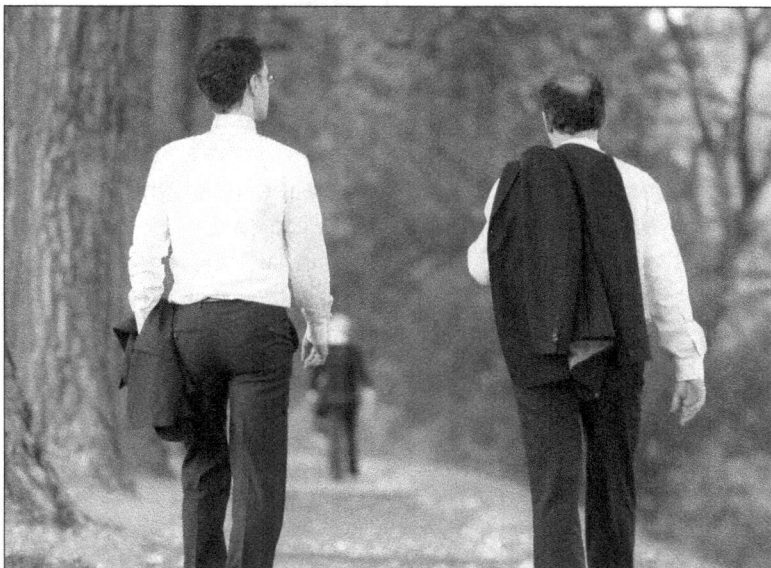

Chapter 7

Getting Rid of your Excess Adrenaline

Is exercise a dirty word?

A little effort goes a long way

In Chapter 4 we discussed the vitally important role that your amygdala plays in the fight or flight response. It is part of your mammal or emotional brain. When the amygdala gets stuck in the "on" position through too many negative thoughts, it is producing adrenaline a great deal of the time. Your anxious thoughts are creating false fight or flight situations and, because you do not have to attack your attacker, defend yourself or run away, the adrenaline produced is hanging around in your body as a toxin. You need to get rid of it.

I realise that "exercise" is a dirty word to some people and certainly going to the gym is not everyone's idea of fun. I fully understand that if you are feeling tired and lethargic you may well not want to go for a jog and if you have ME or CFS you may well be incapable of jogging and might not feel like doing anything at all. However, a little bit of cardiovascular exercise in your office or your home **will** help you get rid of some latent adrenaline and that will combat your tiredness.

Exercise 3

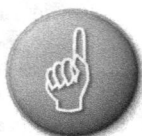

Before doing any exercise it is a good idea to do some basic stretching

Try doing 20 star jumps, or jumping jacks. That should be just enough to use up some of your toxins without exhausting you and without taking up masses of your work time.

You could also try 20 sit ups or 20 push ups if you like that type of exercise, or 20 seconds of running on the spot punching your arms and hands in the air, or 20 seconds of running up the stairs.

20 of anything that gets you moving and burns off a little of the latent adrenalin will make you feel much better and, over a period of time, this will definitely reduce your toxin levels.

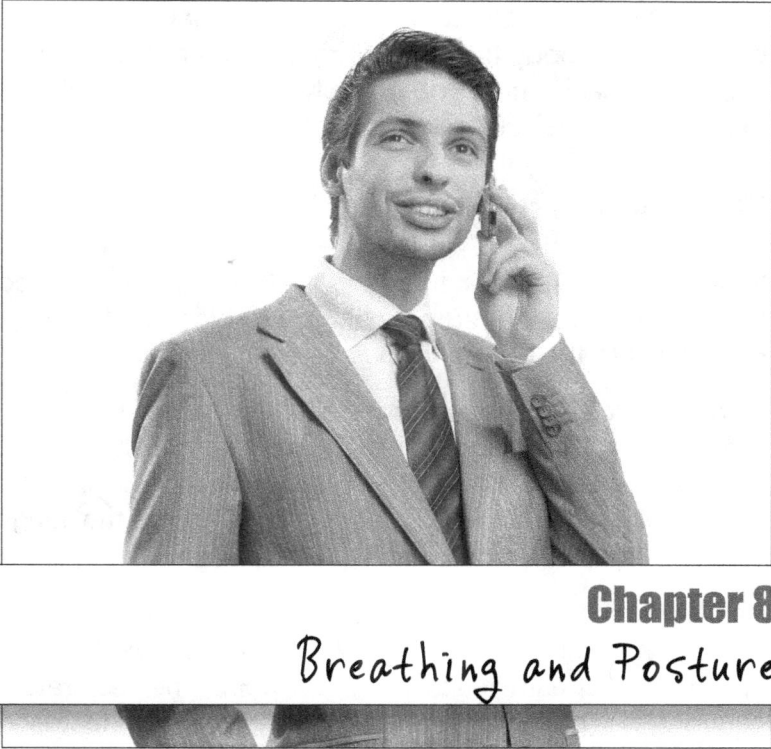

Chapter 8

Breathing and Posture

Every breath you take can make a difference

Breathing

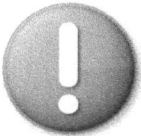

> **You can survive several days without food and water but only a few minutes without air**

Your health depends not only on the quality of the air you breathe but also on how you actually breathe it. It is very easy to fall into bad breathing habits without even realising it. During times of anxiousness, whether perceived or real, our reptilian brain will instruct the body to take shallower quicker breaths. If the body then goes into the fight or flight mode, this can escalate until you actually suffer hyperventilation during a panic attack.

The science of breathing

When we inhale, oxygen travels to the lungs and is collected by haemoglobin (the red pigment inside blood cells) which release it into the body's tissues where it is needed.

Our tissue cells use oxygen in all their energy reactions, producing carbon dioxide and water as a result. Carbon dioxide is needed for every metabolic process and the excess is carried in the bloodstream back to the lungs where it is exhaled along with water vapour.

Carbon dioxide is the main regulator of respiration, controlling the rate & depth of breathing. When carbon dioxide levels in the bloodstream reach a certain point, the respiratory centre in our brain sends a message to the muscles used for breathing to take in more air and breathe out excess carbon dioxide.

If the carbon dioxide levels are low then the haemoglobin will not release the oxygen to the cells. If you are breathing in and out very rapidly you are actually getting less oxygen to the cells that need it, in severe cases this can cause spasms as the muscles of the airways constrict.

Correcting poor breathing techniques is a little like correcting negative thinking. At first you will have to make a conscious effort to make it happen but then, after practice, the reptilian brain and your autonomic nervous system will take over and correct breathing will become the norm for you.

Exercise 4

This exercise is great for correcting your shallow, anxious breathing habits and giving your cells the oxygen that they need.

Breathe in through your nose for the count of three and then breathe out through your mouth slowly for the count of six. It is the breathing out that relaxes you.

Exercise 5

This exercise will build on the stop technique in chapter 6

First of all say aloud the word "STOP" and stop thinking about anything that is making you feel stressed. Live in the now and take a long slow breath in through your nose, hold it for a few seconds and then breathe out through your mouth taking twice as long as when you breathed in. It is important that you control the speed at which you exhale, make sure you take twice as long to exhale as inhale, and remember that it is the exhaling that calms you down.

As you exhale think about the tension in your muscles, allow your back muscles to relax and your stomach muscles to relax allow all the muscles in your arms and legs to relax and all your facial muscles to relax.

Now concentrate on living in the now, think about everything that is happening around you, the light in the room, the smell, what you can see. Really concentrate on them and exclude all other thoughts.

Correct posture

Correct posture and good breathing are very closely linked. There is a common misconception that correct posture means standing or sitting up very straight with your shoulders thrown back. Wrong, this merely tenses your lower back and leg muscles and makes you rigid so restricting your rib cage and inhibiting your breathing.

Correct posture means sitting or standing upright but not tense, being relaxed in your body but not slouching. You could sum it up as, sit or stand up but don't force yourself up.

Exercise 6

This exercise will help both your breathing and your posture.

Sit comfortably in a straight backed chair. Make sure you are relaxed and that you feel warm. Practice living in the now to get rid of any anxious thoughts that you might have and really concentrate on your surroundings. Close your eyes.

Place both of your hands on your stomach and start to imagine that you are growing taller. Really concentrate on growing taller, allow your spine to come straight and grow a few inches. Do not tense your back, do not tense any muscles in your body, just feel it come straight.

Now take a deep breath in to the count of three making sure that your breath is going deep enough to raise your hands on your stomach. Hold the breath for a couple of seconds and then slowly exhale to the count of six as before. Repeat this exercise several times a day and it will start to become an automatic habit.

Exercise 7

This exercise builds on exercise 6 and gives you even more opportunity to relax your muscles.

Stand up with a straight back and your legs shoulder width apart. Now inhale to the count of three like before, but as you do so, raise your arms slowly and rise on to tiptoe simultaneously. As you reach three you should reach the maximum height of your stretch. Hold for two counts and exhale for the count of six. As you exhale drop your arms slowly, and drop down from your toes back to your flat feet.

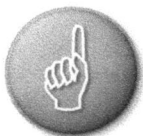

Your mind will not be calm if your body is tense. Concentrate on living in the now to ensure that you are relaxed when you do these exercises.

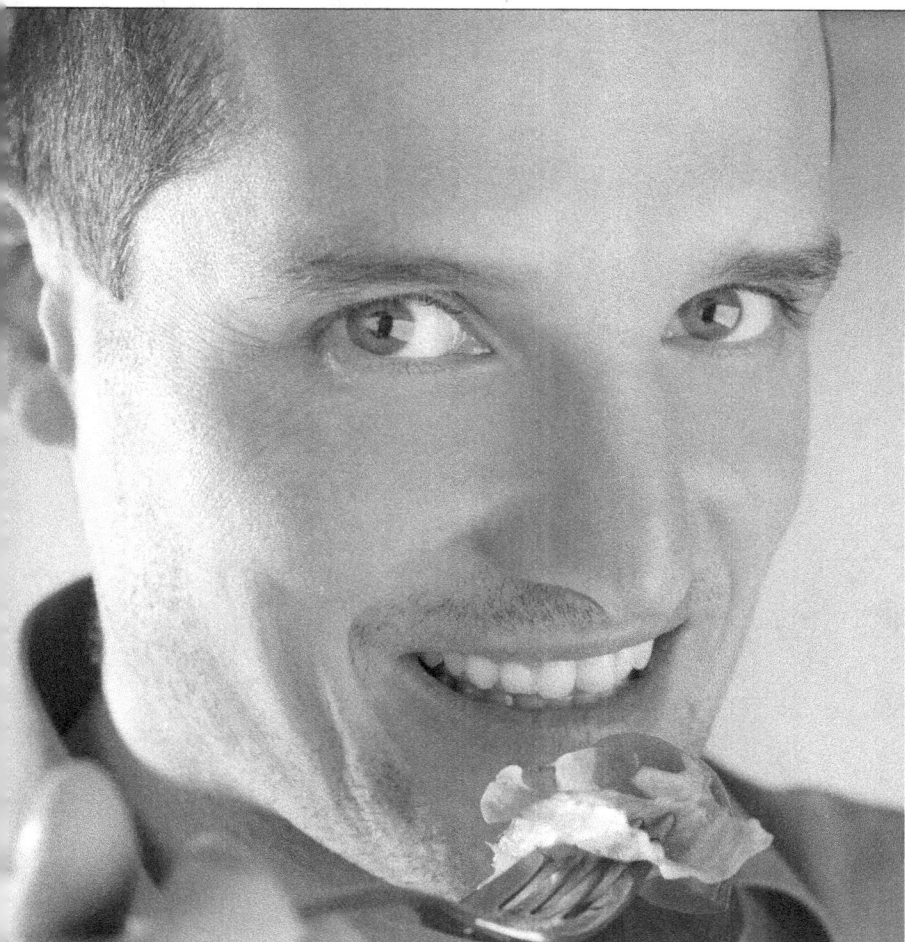

Part 2
It's Always the Right Time to do the Right Thing

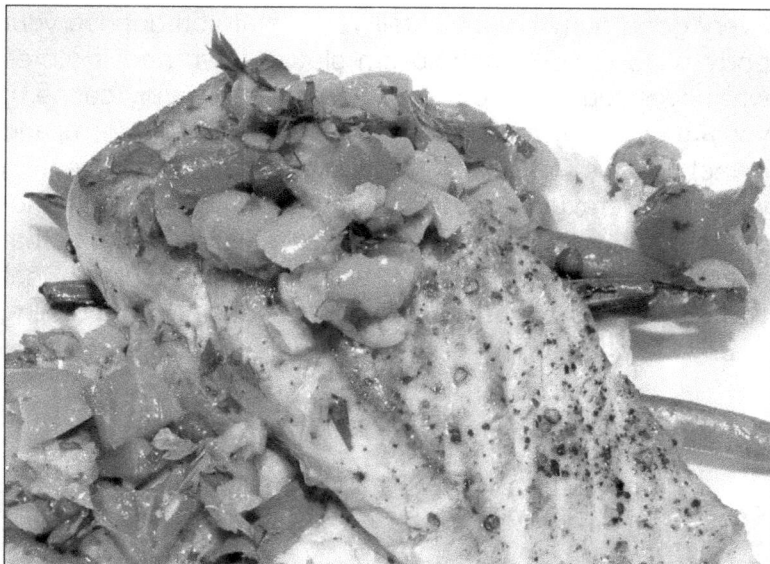

Chapter 9
Your body and food

We are what we eat

We have discussed how your mind has a huge influence on your body, and the opposite is also true. A body full of toxins is a body that is tired and lethargic and a body that is drawing on your mental strength just to keep it fit 4 work and fit 4 life. A body full of toxins is a body that is most likely to be suffering from dis-ease.

Not a diet plan – a life plan

Your body constantly needs fuel to function at its best. It does you no good to go long periods without sustenance.

Every good nutritionist will tell you that if you deprive your body of food your metabolism slows down and it stores what ever you do give it as a sort of emergency cache. If you are trying to, you don't lose weight in the long term, and in fact you are more likely to gain weight from binge eating when your cravings get too much for you. This plan is not about cutting down on food, it is about eating in a way that can make you well. This plan will show you a system that you can use to eat as long as you need to without feeling deprived and without missing out on things that you like.

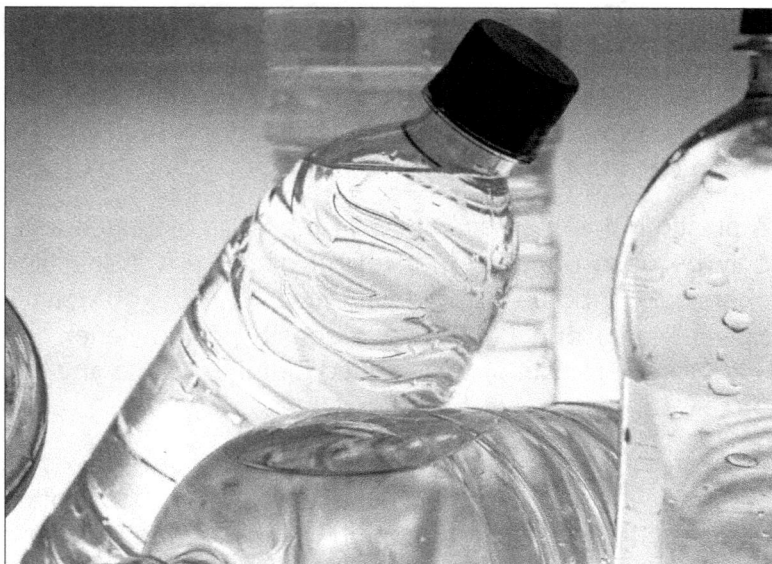

Chapter 10
The Curse of the 3 Ps

Production, preparation and packaging

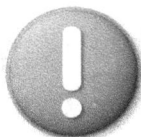

Most modern food production, preparation, and packaging is not kind to your food and not kind to your body.

Manufacturers produce food by growing it using vast amounts of chemical fertilizer, they then process it, adding more chemicals to preserve it, or alter the taste, and they package it, often in plastic – plastic is a chemical product.

Be aware that even a completely pure natural product like spring water can be contaminated by the 3Ps.

Plastic water bottles are known to leach a chemical called Bisphenol A or BPA. This has been linked to breast and uterine cancer in women and decreased testosterone levels in men and can be particularly devastating to babies and young children.

A plastic bottle marked with a #1 recycling symbol should only be used once, do not refill it because it is leaching chemicals, a bottle marked with a #2 HDPE (high density polyethylene), or a #4 LDPE (low density polyethylene), or a #5 PP (polypropylene), is designed for multiple use and can be refilled.

It is not only plastic that you need to be careful of, the 3 Ps are everywhere, for example even recycled cardboard often contains chemicals like Disobutyl phthalate, DIBP, which is found in inks. It can often be present in recycled food packaging if the pulp material contained lots of print.

Personal care products are cursed by the 3Ps

In addition to what we are actually putting into our bodies we need to be aware of what we are putting onto them. Your skin is absorbent, what you put on top of it will find its way into your system.

Most brand name personal care products contain chemicals

Just about every major personal care product brand contains chemicals. For example many leading brands of shampoo contain methylisothiazoline or MIT which has been linked with neurological damage, and contributes in part to Alzheimer's disease and cancer.

Be aware

If you are having a reaction to a particular personal care product, have a look at the label, maybe there is a chemical in there that is having a particular effect on you.

Obviously, in modern life not all chemicals can be avoided and of course our bodies and minds are initially pretty robust, they can take a fair bit of abuse, what is important is to be aware of what you are using and to be aware that if your mind and body are overloaded and have already broken down, then you will have to be especially careful and avoid eating, drinking or using products that are unnecessarily full of toxins.

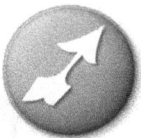

If you buy water in a plastic bottle with a #1 sign and do not finish it all, decant it into a glass bottle for future use. You can refill a glass bottle as often as you wish. I keep a glass bottle in the fridge and fill it and take it with me each day.

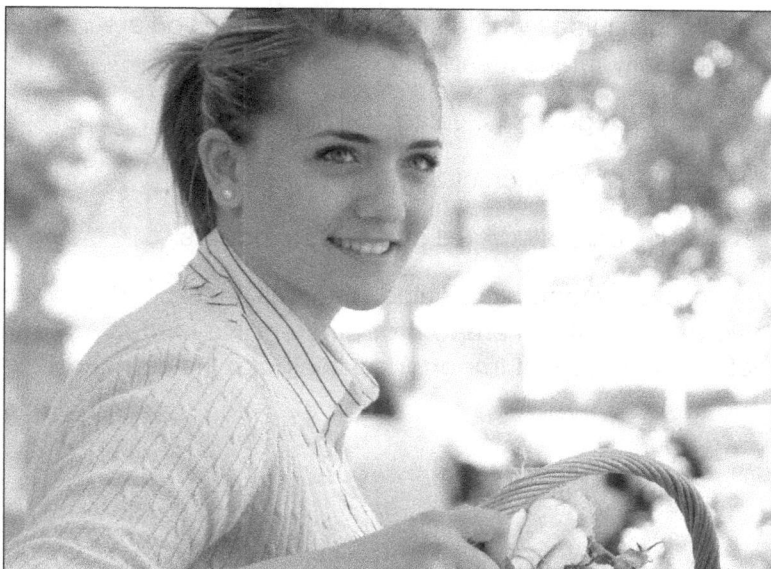

Chapter 11
Eat Yourself Well

Food creates energy

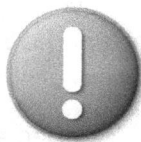

No food is bad for a healthy body if eaten in the right quantities and as part of a balanced diet. The problems occur when your body is overloaded with toxins.

Good, fresh food with a minimum of toxins eaten at regular intervals will help your body and mind to recover from a toxin overload and make you feel full of energy and vitality.

As a rough guide I would suggest that when you are looking at your daily intake it should consist of:

60% vegetables, salad and fruit

20% protein, chicken, turkey or fish

20% carbohydrates and grain products

If you hate vegetables, salad and fruit take heart, do not give up here, there are lots of different ways that you can eat them and, most importantly, it is not a life sentence.

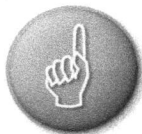 **Not a life sentence**

In the plan the foods are initially split into Yes Foods and No Go Foods

Many people who have followed the plan live by it for the rest of their lives. However, for those of us who hate the sound of No Go Areas, remember, the guidelines here are NOT a life sentence, as soon as you have given your body time to rebalance you can introduce foods from the No-Go list, in small quantities at first then as you please. Obviously, what you can't do is throw all the guidelines away and hope to maintain your improved energy levels.

Naturally if you are already consulting a doctor for special dietary requirements please discuss this plan with them before making any major changes to your daily food intake.

The rules

To eat yourself well there are only 2 rules

Rule 1

Cut out as many additives, E numbers and chemicals as you can.

Rule 2

Rotate your food.

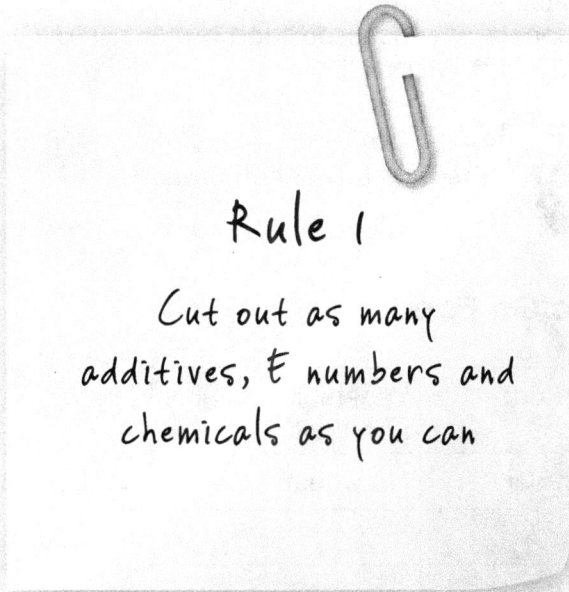

Rule 1

Cut out as many additives, E numbers and chemicals as you can

Eat as much "straight" food as possible.

By "straight" I mean fresh food that has not undergone any processing.

Buy your vegetables from wherever is most convenient, either the farm shop or the supermarket, but buy them as whole foods, not pre stuffed, partly prepared or mashed, and buy them fresh if you possibly can. Obviously cost and convenience is a factor in any diet and frozen food is often much cheaper than fresh, but be careful to check the label for any unwanted additives. If you have to take something from a tin then be aware of what else is in the tin, for example use tinned tuna in brine not in sunflower oil and make sure there is no added sugar in the water. Do not make eating out of a tin a daily habit, treat it as your last resort, not your first call.

Cutting out all additives E numbers and chemicals is not a life sentence – as you get better you will be able to introduce small amounts of processed food but DO NOT CHEAT IN THE FIRST FEW MONTHS.

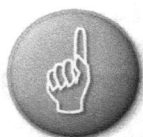

Fresh is best at all times

The No Go Foods

Fish or Meat	Vegetables, Grains and Fruit	Drinks
No red meat	No wheat	No alcohol
No pork		No caffeine
No dairy		No added sugar
No processed foods or added sugar		

Don't be alarmed! There are only 6 food categories on this list and 2 drink categories. This is not a life sentence and the benefits are worth it.

The Yes Foods

Everything else!

To give you a guide.....

Fish or Meat	Vegetables Grains and Fruit	Drinks
Fresh fish all varieties	Fresh vegetables all types	Mineral water
Fresh shellfish all varieties	Fresh fruit all types	Fruit teas
Fresh chicken in moderation	Nuts	Herbal teas
Fresh turkey in moderation	Pulses	Caffeine free tea in moderation
Any other fresh poultry in moderation	Grains	Caffeine free coffee in moderation
		Vegetable juice
		Fruit Juice (dilute with mineral water from a glass bottle)

Why No Go foods?

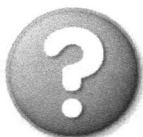

No Alcohol – Why?

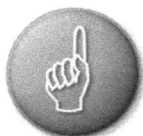

Back to work back to the bottle – 42% of people admit to drinking because of stress.

Commonly people drink alcohol because they think it is a stimulant, that it makes them feel better and more able to cope.

Alcohol is a depressant. It affects your central nervous system. Although the initial effects may seem stimulating, cumulatively it slows down the way you think, speak, move and react.

People think that they can sober up quickly if they need to by having a shower, or coffee or food.

None of these things will make you sober. Only time will remove alcohol from your system; depending on your weight, it takes about one hour to eliminate one unit of alcohol.

Another common misconception is that your body develops a tolerance to alcohol if you drink a lot regularly, so you can safely drink more.

The more you drink the more damage your body will sustain and the greater the risks become. Tolerance is actually a warning sign that your body has started to be affected by alcohol.

A bottle of wine (ABV 13.5%) contains 10 units of alcohol. Current medical evidence endorses the fact that the recommended daily limit guidelines are 3 - 4 units for men and 2 - 3 units for women. So, sharing a daily bottle of wine with a partner puts both of you over the recommended limit for each day.

Around 10 million people in the UK regularly drink more than half a bottle of wine a day. Regularly exceeding the guidelines increases the risk of long-term health problems.

Since 1979 alcohol-related deaths have almost tripled among men and almost doubled among women.

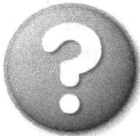

No Caffeine - Why?

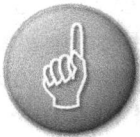

Caffeine is the most widely used drug in the world, just one small cup of brewed coffee contains between 80 – 115 mg of caffeine. Tea has roughly half that amount as does a typical soda soft drink.

Caffeine stimulates the central nervous system and it can cause heightened anxiety and body tension - stress - just the thing that you are trying to avoid.

Caffeine does not give you energy. Scientifically, it is not possible to measure any increase in energy provided by caffeine. It is a mind enhancing drug that makes you more alert and raises your stress levels as evidenced in tests by spikes in stress hormones, elevations in blood pressure and heart rate, but no one would claim that these are positive benefits.

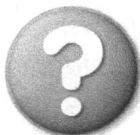

No Wheat - Why?

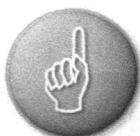

Wheat is the most difficult of all the grains to digest. Most people do not absorb a large amount of the starch in wheat. These starches get fermented by the bacteria in the digestive system, which then produce acids which damage the lining of your system letting toxins leak into your blood.

Wheat is a relatively new food for the human race. Ancient man did not cultivate it. Cultivation of wheat and other grains started around 12,000 years ago and genetic testing has discovered that many people have simply not adapted to the introduction of wheat into the diet.

Wheat contains gluten, a family of proteins, that as many as one in three people may be sensitive to, and, in the refining process chemical preservatives are added to extend its shelf life.

Note: gluten is also found in rye, barley and oats but it is a different type and can be tolerated by many people who react to wheat gluten.

Your digestive system provides a barrier between the foods you eat and your blood stream but if this barrier breaks down gliadin, one of the two main proteins in gluten, gets into the blood stream. The immune system reacts to it and it becomes a toxin.

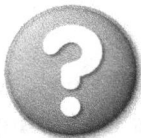

No Dairy - Why?

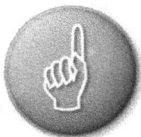

Dairy is another group of products that are difficult for the body to cope with.

Once you are weaned, as many as 75% of people lose the ability to digest lactose, which is a milk sugar.

Lactose intolerance can cause gastric upset which in turn can cause the digestive barrier to break down which places a heavy load on the liver detox system.

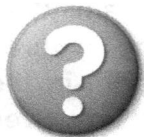

No Red Meat - Why?

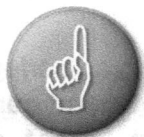

Many animals are injected with antibiotics, hormones and chemicals that make them grow fast and large. When we consume meat we also consume these chemicals.

Tumour and cancer cells in animals can cause tumour and cancer cells in humans.

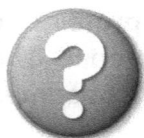

No Pork – Why?

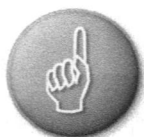

No ham, sausages, salami or cured meat.

Pork, in the majority of its forms, tends to have more fat than other meats and many E numbers are used in its curing.

Pigs are scavengers and eat a wide range of rotting and unhealthy foods. They have a similar immune system to our own which means that several diseases are easily transferrable between them and us.

A pig's respiratory tract is receptive to both human and bird flu viruses so it can act as a breeding ground for really unpleasant viruses.

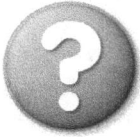

Limited Sugar – Why?

This includes limited honey.

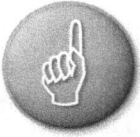

Sugar intake causes our blood sugars to rise in a rush and then afterwards we suffer the down. When this happens, the body releases hormones to bring the sugar level in our blood back to our optimum level, these hormones include adrenaline, cortisol and epinephrine – the stress hormones that put us back into the fight or flight mode.

Fluctuating blood sugar levels leads to feelings of fatigue and exhaustion.

Too much sugar can weaken your immune system. Excess sugar in the blood causes the incumbent bacteria and yeast to multiply and if they get to high levels they can weaken the immune system.

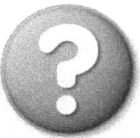

No Processed Food - Junk – Why?

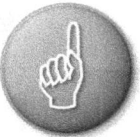

What happens when you feed kids junk food? - They go hyper.

Processed food is full of E numbers and additives.

Why Yes Foods?

The most important aid to recovery is water. **Mineral water,** ideally from a glass bottle so that you avoid the chemicals inherent in the plastic. Your body is 60% water, it is important that you keep that topped up every day, lots of people spend most of their life dehydrated and this puts a strain on their bodies. If you are actually feeling thirsty, you are already dehydrated. Drink at least 2 – 3 litres of mineral water a day – go on drink to your own health!

Fresh vegetables – eat these raw or only minimally cooked.

Fresh vegetables are full of vitamins and minerals and are good sources of dietary fibre. They're naturally low in fat, sodium and calories and contain no cholesterol. They **are** good for you. In addition many have natural substances called phytochemicals which actually help prevent some conditions like diabetes, and some cancers. Vegetables with high phytochemicals include tomatoes, broccoli, beans, peas and lentils. Many vegetables are also high in antioxidants which are the substances that slow down cell damage so in simple terms can reduce the ageing process. If you think that you don't like vegetables, try lots of different types, there will be some that you find you enjoy, and eat them in different ways, you might hate boiled carrots but like them raw for instance.

All vegetables are included in the plan but avoid eating large quantities of the ones that are full of oil, like avocados, and when having potatoes eat them boiled or baked NOT FRIED, also avoid fried aubergine as it soaks up the oil when you cook it.

Fresh fruit – eat this raw or baked.

Fresh fruit like vegetables is full of vitamins and is virtually cholesterol free. It too can prevent heart diseases and some cancers and it can improve your memory. Fruit has a very high water content so it is easily absorbed by the body which means the goodness can get to the right places quickly. Again if you think you don't like fruit, be brave, try lots of different types, there will be something that you enjoy.

Every kind of fruit is included in the plan but beware of the sugar content – Bananas are really high in fructose (sugar) and so are grapes. Dried fruit needs to be eaten in small quantities too because it has much more sugar than fresh.

(See fructose table below)

Nuts – in moderation, around a couple of ounces a day.

At the Loma Linda University in California a study done in the 1990s showed that people eating nuts every day had up to 60% fewer heart attacks than those who ate nuts less than once per month. Try taking some nuts with you as a snack. Again try all types of nuts if it is a foodstuff that you don't normally eat, they have wide ranging flavours and textures and there will be one that you like.

All nuts are included in the plan but be aware that peanuts are very high in oil.

All fresh fish – eat more of the white non-oily fish like plaice, cod, halibut or sea bass and less of the oily fish like salmon or tuna.

Fresh fish is high in omega 3 fatty acids that help prevent heart disease and fish is high in protein and low in fat. There are so many fish families that you can eat it every day if you want to.

Don't be tempted to eat much smoked fish – the processing, smoking and packaging nearly always contains a preservative!

All shellfish – crustaceans and molluscs including: oysters, mussels, clams, crabs, scallops, shrimp or prawns and lobster.

Shellfish often has a bad name, in the ocean crustaceans and molluscs naturally ingest or filter organisms and, if the water is contaminated, they can ingest bacteria and viruses. Be sure you are buying your shellfish from an approved source and do not eat it raw, the bacteria is killed in the cooking process.

Shellfish is high in protein and low in fat, cooked properly it is delicious but just be sensible, if it doesn't agree with you leave it out, there is plenty else in the plan to chose from.

Chicken and turkey – Organic and in moderation.

Chicken and turkey are both high in protein and low in fat, in fact they are the leanest meats available and contain B vitamins, Zinc and selenium.

Don't be tempted to buy super cheap chicken, be sure of your source because very cheap chicken may well have been injected with extra water and e numbers.

Pulses – There is a really wide variety, for example lentils, beans and chickpeas.

Again pulses are a great source of protein and studies have shown that they reduce the risk of heart disease. In one study it was found that 69 - 200 gms of pulses per day reduced blood cholesterol level by 10%

All pulses are included, but watch the sugar content. (See fructose table in Chapter 12)

Grains - rice, millet, oats, barley and rye but eat the whole grain rather than the refined grain if you can.

There is compelling evidence to show that whole grains can reduce heart disease and some cancers.

All grains EXCEPT WHEAT

Drink

Mineral water from a glass bottle – this should be by far your most frequent drink. If you want other drinks then those listed below can be taken in moderation:

Fruit teas

Herbal teas

Vegetable juice

Fruit juice - watered down (with mineral water).

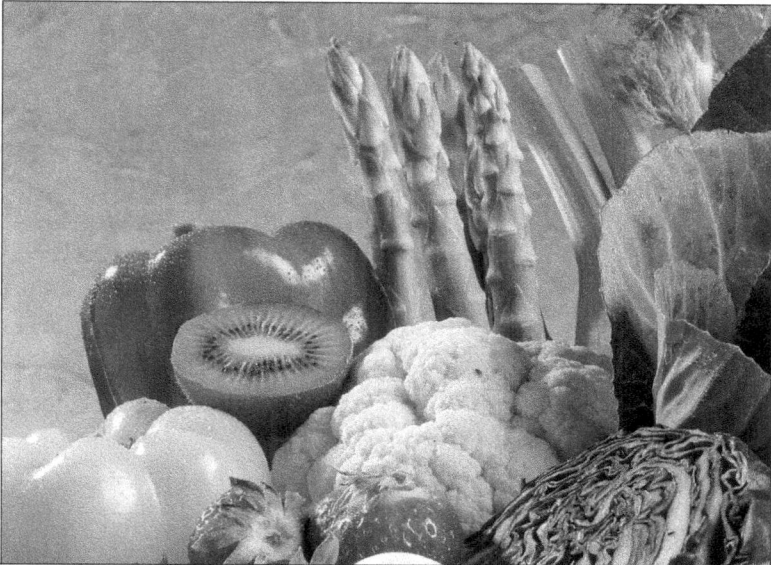

Chapter 12
Fructose

All fruit, nuts and vegetables contain fructose, it is a natural form of sugar. Use the table to make sure that you eat more of the fruit, nuts and vegetables that have a low fructose content and limit the intake of the ones that are high. You can inadvertently give yourself a sugar rush, and consequently suffer the downside, if you eat too much dried fruit for example.

Fructose (SUGAR) table (alphabetical)

Fruit and Nuts

Very Low	Low	Medium	High
Almonds	Apricots	Apples	Bananas
Brazil nuts	Blackberries	Apricots (dried)	Currants
Coconuts	Damsons	Chestnuts	Figs (dried)
Cranberries	Figs (green)	Grapes (black)	Peaches (dried)
Gooseberries	Grapefruit	Grapes (white)	Prunes (dried)
Lemons	Greengages	Melons (yellow)	Raisins
Loganberries	Mandarins	Nectarines	Sultanas (dried)
Melons	Medlars	Peaches	
Rhubarb	Mulberries	Pears	
Walnuts	Oranges	Pineapple	
	Passion fruit	Plums	
	Quinces	Pomegranate	
	Raspberries		
	Tangerines		

Vegetables

Very Low		Low	Medium	High
Asparagus	Artichokes	Beans broad	Beetroot	Lentils (dried)
Broccoli	Avocado	Leeks	Horseradish	Peas (dried)
Cabbage	Beans (French)	Mustard and cress	Parsnips	
Cauliflower	Carrots	Onions	Peas	
Chicory	Celery		Potatoes	
Egg plant	Cucumber	Radishes	Yams	
Marrow	Lettuce	Sweet potatoes		
Pumpkin	Mushroom			
Salsify	Radish			
Sprouts	Spinach			
Tomatoes	Swede			
Watercress	Turnips			

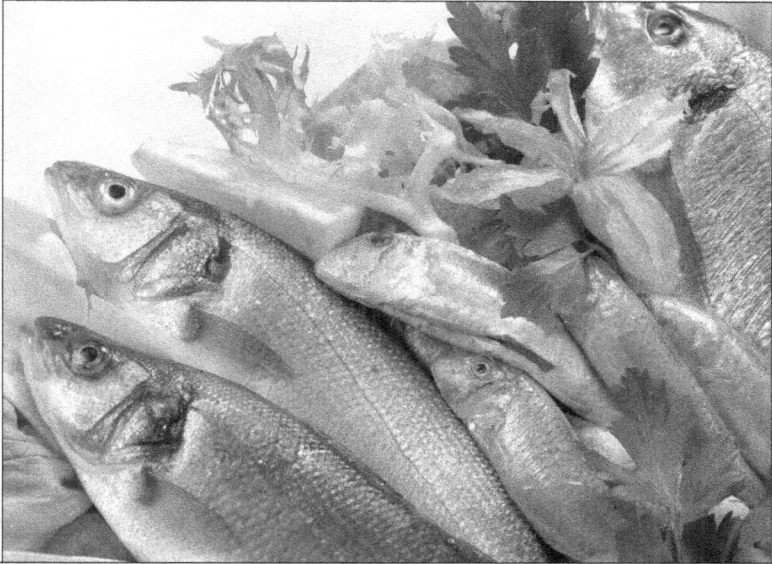

Chapter 13

Rotate Your Food

When you eat your food is just as important as what you eat

Rule 2

Rotate your food

Food rotation

There are two golden rules for food rotation.

1 Eat a certain type of food only every 5 days i.e. if you eat apples on Monday you cannot eat them again until Friday.

2 Eat foods in their respective families for e.g. potatoes, capsicum (peppers) and tomatoes are all in the same family. If you eat potatoes on Monday you may as well eat a meal that contains tomatoes and capsicum, if you like these foods, because you cannot eat any of the family until Friday.

In the next section are some clear charts showing the permitted foods and their families. Use the charts as a daily reference to make sure that you only eat a food family every 5 days.

There is no limit to how many different families you can eat in a day, but in the early stages, while you are getting used to the system, it might be easier to limit your families to your favourites and get into a weekly routine.

The rotation diet is at the heart of the recovery programme

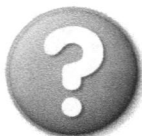

Why rotate food?

It takes 3 days for food to completely clear your system. So, by eating on a 4 day rotation plan, (i.e. eating a specific food only every 5 days) you are allowing your body time to recover from the effects of each particular food and you are preventing a build up of a food that might be upsetting your system.

Remember food rotation and the No Go foods is not a life sentence. In as little as 3 - 6 months you should be able to increase your body's tolerance to a food that was upsetting you and you can then re introduce it in small amounts and slowly – every 10 days and then every 7 then every 5.

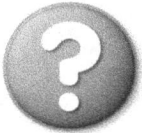

What happens if you don't feel better?

Be careful, every person is different and everybody's reaction is different. When you have sorted out what foods you want to eat on your rotation, you must make sure that they all agree with you. If you do not start to feel better within a couple of weeks, a month at the most, then you need to see if you have an allergic reaction to one of the foods that are still included.

For example you may be eating mussels or prawns that are upsetting you or you may be including a fruit that is high in sugar content and that is upsetting you. If you suspect a food add it for 2 days at a time, if it causes no reaction then fine, continue with it, if it does exclude it.

It is quite normal when your body is overloaded and run down to find that certain foods will have a dramatic effect.

When I was really suffering with M.E. (Myalgic Encephalomyelitis) and was beginning to experiment with the food I ate, I found that when I ate potatoes I was much less mobile than if I had not eaten them. The reaction would come on almost immediately, I would not feel like walking and if I tried I found that the use of my legs was impaired.

Strawberries also had a dramatic effect on me, they made my speech slurred.

The reactions were really frightening and so I excluded these foods, and all other foods in their families for 6 months, and then found that I could eat small amounts of them without suffering any ill effects. Now I eat both foods and all their family groups on my 4 day rotation and do not suffer any problems.

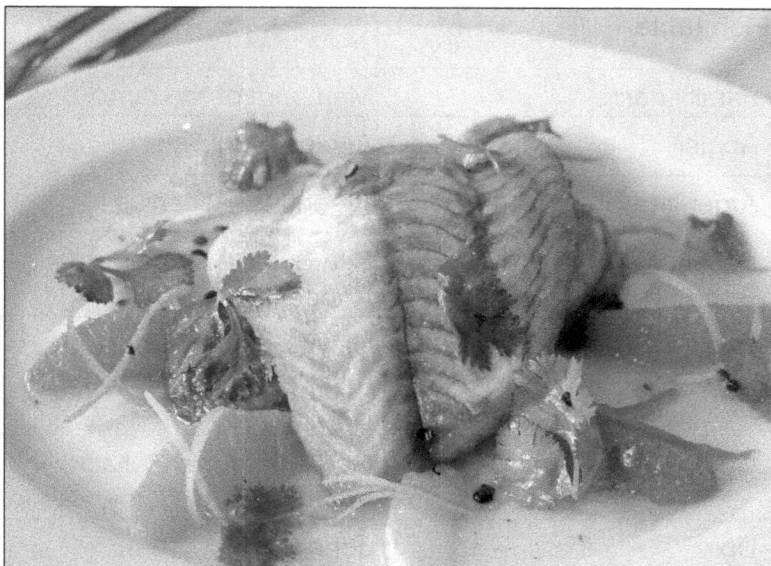

Chapter 14
Foods in Their Families

Your body loves food in the same family

I bought the following table as a poster for £5. It was sponsored by a charity and is probably the best £5 I ever spent on food or food related products. The table covers the most popular foods and foods that are readily available in most countries.

Families are shown in alphabetical order

Fish table

Family name	Members of the family
Angler	Angler, Monkfish
Argentine	Argentine, Ascanius
Bass	Sea Bass, Grouper, Veille Rouge
Carp	Carp, Bream, Gudgeon, Minnow, Orfe, Rudd, Tench, Barble,
Cod	Cod, Haddock, Pollack, Whiting, Pout, Coley, Saithe
Dory	John Dory
Eel	Conger Eel, Eel
Emperor	Red Emperor, Bourgeois
Fresh water Catfish	Fresh Water Catfish
Garfish	Garfish
Grayling	Grayling
Gunnard	Grey Gunnard, Red Gunnard, Yellow Gunnard
Hake	Hake, Burbot, Ling
Herring	Herring, Anchovy, Pilchard, Sardine, Shad, Sprat, Twaite, Whitebait
Lamprey	Lampery, Lampern
Mackerel	Mackerel, Tuna, Bonito
Mullet	Red Mullet

Parrot	Parrotfish
Perch	Perch, Zander
Pike	Pike
Plaice	Plaice, Halibut, Lemon Sole, Dab, Flounder
Salmon	Salmon, Brown Trout, Rainbow Trout
Scad	Scad
Scorpion	Scorpion Fish, Redfish
Sea Catfish	Rock Salmon, Catfish, Rockfish
Seabream	Red Seabream, Bogue
Shark	Shark
Skate	Skate
Snapper	Red Snapper, Grey Snapper
Sole	Dover Sole, Thick Backed Sole
Swordfish	Swordfish
Turbot	Turbot, Brill, Megrim

Shellfish table

Family name	Members of the family
Crustacean	Crab, Lobster, Prawn, Crayfish, Langoustine, Scampi, Shrimp

Mollusc table

Family name	Members of the family
Mollusc	Abalone, Clam, Cockle, Mussel, Oyster, Scallop, Squid, Whelk, Winkle

Fowl table

Family name	Members of the family
Duck	Duck, Duck Eggs
Pheasant	Chicken, Hens Eggs, Pheasant
Turkey	Turkey, Turkey Eggs

Vegetable table

Family name	Members of the family
Avocado	Avocado
Beet	Beetroot, Spinach, Quinoa, Swiss Chard
Caper	Caper
Carrot	Carrot, Celery, Celeriac, Fennel, Parsnip
Cotton	Okra
Fig	Breadfruit, Jack Fruit, Hop Shoots,
Fungi	Mushroom, Truffle,
Gourd	Bitter Gourd, Bottle Gourd, Calabash, Courgette, Cucumber, Gherkin, Gourd, Marrow, Pumpkin, Squash

Lily	Asparagus, Leek, Lnion, Shallot, Spring Onion, Garlic
Mint	Chinese And Japanese Artichoke
Mustard	Cauliflower, Broccoli, Brussels Sprouts, Cabbage, Chinese Leaves, Cress, Radish, Rocket, Swede, Turnip, Watercress
Olive	Olive
Palm	Coconut, Palm Cabbage
Pea	Garden Peas, Split Red Peas, Split Peas, Chick Peas, Snap Peas Mange Tout, Lentil, Alfalfa, Adzuki Bean Sprouts and all types of beans eg Black Beans, Butter Beans, Cannelloni Beans, Cluster Beans, Flageolet Beans, French Beans, Green Beans, Runner Beans String Beans, Haricot Beans, Hyacinth Beans, Jack Beans Kidney Beans, Lima Beans, Mung Beans, Pinto Beans, Soya Beans
Potato	Potato, Tomato, Capsicum (Peppers), Chilli, Aubergine
Reed	Chinese Water Chestnut, Scirpus, Tuberosus
Sunflower	Lettuce, Chicory, Dandelion, Endive, Globe Artichoke, Jerusalem Artichoke, Salsify

Fruit table

Family name	Members of the family
Banana	Banana, Plantain
Berry Rose	Strawberry, Raspberry, Loganberry, Blackberry
Buckwheat	Rhubarb
Carambola	Carambola, Starfruit
Cashew	Mango
Citrus	Orange, Grapefruit, Lemon, Lime
Clove	Guava, Brazil Cherry
Currant	Blackcurrant, Gooseberry, Redcurrant,
Dillenia	Kiwi
Fig	Fig, Hop, Mulberry
Gourd	Melon
Grape	Grape, Rasin, Sultana
Palm	Date
Papaya	Papaya
Passionflower	Passion Fruit
Pineapple	Pineapple
Pome Rose	Apple, Pear
Potato	Tree Tomato, Cape Gooseberry, Naranjilla, Pepino, Lulita, Lulo
Prunus Rose	Peach, Nectarine, Plum, Cherry, Damson, Apricot

Saxifrage	Gooseberry, Blackcurrant, Redcurrant, White Currant
Soapberry	Lychee

Nut and seed table

Family name	Members of the family
Brazil	Brazil, Para, Paradise, Supucaia
Conifer	Pinenut
Gourd	Marrow Seed, Oysternuts, Pumpkin Seed
Grass	Popcorn
Hazel	Cobut, Filbert, Hazelnut
Mango	Chashew, Dhobis, Pistachio
Palm	Coconut
Pea	Groundnut, Monkey, Peanut,
Protea	Macadamia
Prunus rose	Almond
Reed	Tiger, Chufa, Earth Almond, Rush
Sesame	Sesame Seeds
Sunflower	Sunflower Seed
Sweet chestnut	Chestnut,
Walnut	Hickory, Pecan, Walnut

Drinks table

Note: All fruit and vegetables can be taken as drinks as above but dilute to taste if there is a high fructose content.

Family name	Members of the family
Carrot	Fennel
Clove	Eucalyptus
Cocoa	Chocolate, Cocoa
Cotton	Hibiscus
Forget-me-not	Borage, Comfrey
Ginseng	Ginseng
Grass	Barley, Malt
Honeysuckle	Elder Flower
Lime	Linden Flower, Lime Blossom
Madder	Quinine
Mint	Catnip, Hyssop, Lavender, Lemon Balm, Peppermint, Rosemary
Nettle	Nettle
Olive	Jasmine
Pea	Carob, Red Clover
Rose	Rosehip
Sunflower	Burdock, Chamomile, Chicory, Dandelion
Verbena	Lemon Verbena, Verbena

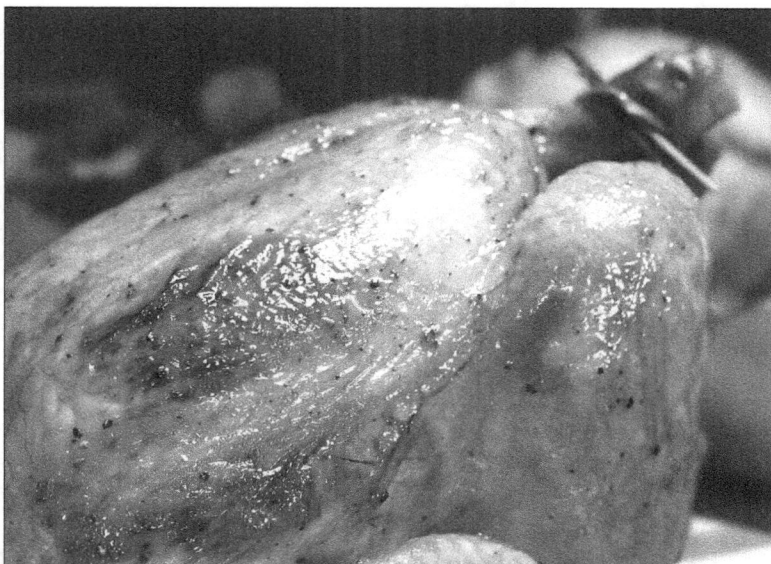

Chapter 15

The Rotation Diet

Food rotation is not limited

This is a really important point, this plan is not about deprivation, it is about eating yourself back to full health. You can eat as much as you want of all the foods on the Yes Foods list, there is a huge variety.

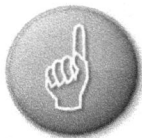

Most people only eat a very limited number of foods and this in part contributes to their feelings of tiredness and lethargy as their body never has a break from them.

Exercise 8

If you are in any doubt about this plan and are wondering if there is enough variety of food for you to eat, write down what you actually *do* eat every day for a week. I think you will be surprised. Most working people tend to have the same sandwich for lunch each day from Monday to Friday, and many people have the same type of food for dinner each night, it might be different varieties of pizza or pasta but it is still pizza and pasta and it might be different chicken dishes but it is still chicken, it might be different varieties of cheese, but it is still cheese.

Getting started

Making life simple - my personal experience

I found that it was easier to get started on the rotation diet and understand it by keeping things very simple for the first few weeks. My health improved immediately and this made it easy to stick to the rotation. I split the foods that I liked, and thought that I could eat regularly, up into day groups so that I could mix and match them. I chose 27 families of food in all. That gave me plenty of variety to prevent me becoming bored but was a number that I could easily deal with and could order in one shop. I actually found a local man who went to the market every day and delivered fruit, vegetables and fish door to door. This had two benefits – I could still eat although I was too debilitated to go out and secondly, it also avoided any temptations in the supermarket if someone else shopped for me and tried to be "kind" and bring me a "treat". If you do not have a local delivery guy and are too debilitated to get out, use the internet or ask a friend to help but make sure you give them a definitive list.

First steps to understanding the rotation diet

Keep it simple.

I chose 4 families of fish that I liked and allotted one to each day of my rotation.

I chose 8 families of vegetables that I liked.

I chose 9 families of fruit that I liked.

I chose 5 types of nuts that I liked.

I chose only 1 cereal that I liked because I did not particularly like cereal.

I quickly learnt all the members of each food family that I liked and started creating some recipes. By approaching it in this way I found that I did not have to keep referring to the charts and giving myself a headache working out what I could eat.

As soon as I had the hang of the rotation I expanded my food groups.

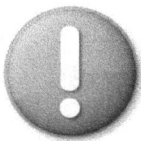

When you chose a family, you do not have to eat every member of it if you do not like a particular food. For example I chose the pea family but did not particularly like lentils so I didn't eat them, there were plenty of other members of the family that I did enjoy.

Fish

(note: I had cut out chicken and turkey for the first 3 months)

Family	Fish
Plaice	Plaice
Cod	Cod and Haddock
Mackerel	Mackerel and Tuna
Crustacean	Shellfish

Vegetables

Family	Vegetable
Lily	Asparagus, Leek and Onion
Carrot	Carrot and Parsnip
Mustard	Cabbage, Cauliflower and Broccoli
Potato	Potato, Tomato and Capsicum (peppers)
Gourd	Courgette and Cucumber
Sunflower	Lettuce and Artichoke
Fungi	Mushrooms
Pea	Peas and Beans, all types

Fruit

Family	Fruit
Pome rose	Apples and Pears
Citrus	Oranges, grapefruit and Lemons

Actinidia	Kiwi
Mango	Mango
Berry rose	Strawberries, Raspberries, LoganBerries and Blackberries
Gourd	Melon (eat on same day as Courgette and Cucumber)
Banana	Bananas (but not many due to the high sugar content)
Pineapple	Pineapple
Prunus rose	Nectarines, Peaches, Apricots, Plums

Cereal

Family	Cereal
Grass	Oat bran

Nuts and seeds

Family	Nut
Brazil	Brazil nuts
Walnut	Walnuts and Pecan nuts
Hazel	Hazel nuts
Mango	Cashew nuts (eat on the same day as Mangos)
Gourd	Pumpkin seeds, Oyster nuts (eat on same day as Courgettes)

Obviously your choice of foods is personal but my advice is to keep it really simple, decide on foods that you like and can eat for the first couple of weeks while you get used to the system.

Typical 4 day rotation

A typical 4 day rotation using the above ingredients is shown in the table below.

All the recipes can be found in the recipe section.

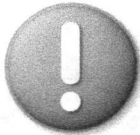

I was working from home much of the time I experimented with this. Obviously some work places have good cooking/heating up facilities and others do not. In the food rotation and work section in chapter 16 there are practical hints and ideas to make eating on rotation with no cooking facilities feasible and enjoyable.

Day 1

	Menu	Recipe	Families
Breakfast	Bananas and brazil nuts		Banana Brazil
Lunch	Grilled Plaice with rosemary and garlic, serve with boiled asparagus and peas		Plaice Lily Pea
	Exotic fruit salad: Nectarines; Bananas; Apricots; Plums		Prunus rose Banana

Dinner	Microwave steamed fish: Plaice steamed in microwave with onions and ginger Served with boiled asparagus and leeks		Plaice Lilly Ginger
	Baked bananas and nectarines		Banana Prunus rose
Snacks	Brazil nuts Whole Nectarines bananas Plums Apricots Peaches Raw peas in their pods		Brazil Banana Prunus rose Pea
Drinks	Water Diluted nectarine juice Ginseng tea		Ginseng Prunus rose

Day 2

	Menu	Recipe	Families
Breakfast	Oat bran with orange juice		Grass Citrus
Lunch	Lemon and Lime Prawns Serve with lettuce and herb salad		Citrus Crustacean Sunflower mint

Dinner	Brochette of Scallops: Serve with rice and a side salad of lettuce with herbs		Crustacean Pineapple Grass
	Mixed citrus fruit bowl		Citrus
Snacks	Walnuts, pecan nuts Oranges Grapefruit Pineapple		Walnut Citrus Pineapple
Drinks	Water Diluted orange juice Chamomile tea		Citrus Sunflower

Day 3

	Menu	Recipe	Families
Breakfast	Kiwi and strawberries		Actinidia Berry rose
Lunch	Grilled Cod Served with boiled cabbage, cauliflower and broccoli Mixed berry compote		Cod Mustard Berry rose

Dinner	Grilled Haddock Served with carrot and parsnip mash		Cod Carrot
	Mango		Mango
Snacks	Hazel nuts Kiwi Strawberries Raspberries Loganberries Mango Raw carrot Raw broccoli & cauliflower		Hazel Berry rose Mango Mustard
Drinks	Water Diluted mango juice, kiwi juice or strawberry juice Strawberry tea		Actinidia Berry rose Mango

Day 4

	Menu	Recipe	Families
Breakfast	Melon cocktail		Gourd
Lunch	Tuna kebabs and baked aubergine Serve with roasted courgettes Apples Pears		Potato Gourd Mackerel Pome rose

Dinner	Mackerel and courgettes Served with roasted peppers and tomatoes and mushrooms and baked potatoes Honeydew melon		Potato Mackerel Fungi Gourd
Snacks	Pumpkin seeds Oyster nuts Melon Apples Pears		Gourd Pome rose
Drinks	Water Rosehip tea		Pome rose

To make the initial rotation really simple I used all of the fruit and vegetables I had chosen. However, I quickly found that I could manage with less families which gave me a wider rotation choice.

For example:

Day 1	If I only ate bananas as my fruit, that would free up the prunus rose family (plums, apricots, peaches)
Day 2	If I only ate citrus fruits that would free up the pineapple family (pineapple)
Day 3	If I only ate berries that would free up the actinidia family (kiwi)
Day 4	If I only ate melon that would free up the pome rose family (apples and pears)

Just by this simple change it meant I could eat a different fruit family for 8 days. The same applies to the vegetables and of course I did not need to eat fish every day. In this way, my food selection could make up a lot of different meals.

In the next chapter I have made a simple change to the above rotation to adapt it for the workplace where there may be no cooking or heating up facilities.

Cooking essentials

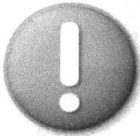

When you cook do not drown your food in fat or oil it is not good for you.

- **Use a spray of oil, using a non aerosol spray to dampen the bottom of the pan.**

- **Use the oven to bake meat and fish – there is no need to add any oil.**

- **Use the grill to cook meat, fish and vegetables and again use no oil or just a spray.**

- **Steam your food with water in the bottom of the steamer. Some of my recipes say use a microwave to steam dishes as opposed to a traditional steamer. I found no health problems using a microwave and it is easier and faster than a steamer particularly if you are at work. I acknowledge that some people may not wish to microwave their food and in that case all the recipes will work well with a traditional steamer.**

- **Use a frying pan with just a spray of oil on the bottom and toss vegetables quickly to just soften them and turn meat/fish quickly to prevent sticking.**

When is strict possibly too strict?

A really strict food rotation would obviously also include the oil and fat that you cooked in, the herbs that you used and every variety of fruit or herbal teal that you drank.

I took the view that all these things were used in such small quantities that I did not necessarily rotate them strictly although I did not have the same one every day. A cooking essential is to only use a spray of oil, herbs are used for flavour and easily available fruit and herbal teas usually have a wide number of fruit ingredients in them but in very small quantities.

I have included their tables in the appendix should you wish to rotate them strictly.

More varied 4 day rotation with chicken and turkey

There are a huge number of foods on the Yes list you can eat in rotation. It is very likely that on this plan you are going to eat a wider variety of foods than before.

An example of a more varied rotation including chicken and turkey is below. Drinks are mineral water and diluted fruit and vegetable juice as per the rotation or herbal or fruit tea.

Day 1	Fish/Meat	Vegetables	Fruit	Nuts/Seeds
Families	Pheasant Herring Crustacean	Pea Sunflower Avocado Fig	Prunus rose Fig Saxifrage Soapberry Pineapple	Pea Prunus rose Sunflower

Day 2	Fish/Meat	Vegetables	Fruit	Nuts/Seeds
Families	Salmon Mackerel Cod	Lily Gourd Olive Cotton	Citrus Pawpaw Grape Papaya Carambola	Walnut Gourd

Day 3	Fish/Meat	Vegetables	Fruit	Nuts/Seeds
Families	Plaice Bass Turkey	Potato Mustard Fungi Grass	Pome rose Currant Banana Palm Potato	Brazil Grass Palm

Day 4	Fish/Meat	Vegetables	Fruit	Nuts/Seeds
Families	Sole Hake Mullet	Carrot Beet Reed Caper	Mango Actinidia Berry rose Buckwheat Pomegranate	Sesame Hazel Mango

Not a diet plan

The primary aim of this plan is to give your body time to recover from its toxins, it is not a diet plan in the sense that it is not specifically designed for weight loss. In reality, many people do find that they lose weight with this eating pattern because they are eating fresh fish and meat, fresh vegetables and fruit rather than packaged foods with lots of added sugar, and salt.

The rotations described above do not have a great deal of bulk in them, I found that suited me best, however if you feel hungry and need more bulk then remember that there are many breads and starches that do not contain wheat and feel free to add these in and rotate them as above. From the grass family try rice cakes and corn cakes and Ryvita (except the one that contains fruit crunch these are all wheat free). From the pea family try chick pea, gram and soya, from the potato family try products with potato flour and try tahini from the sesame family. The flour and starch table is in the appendix.

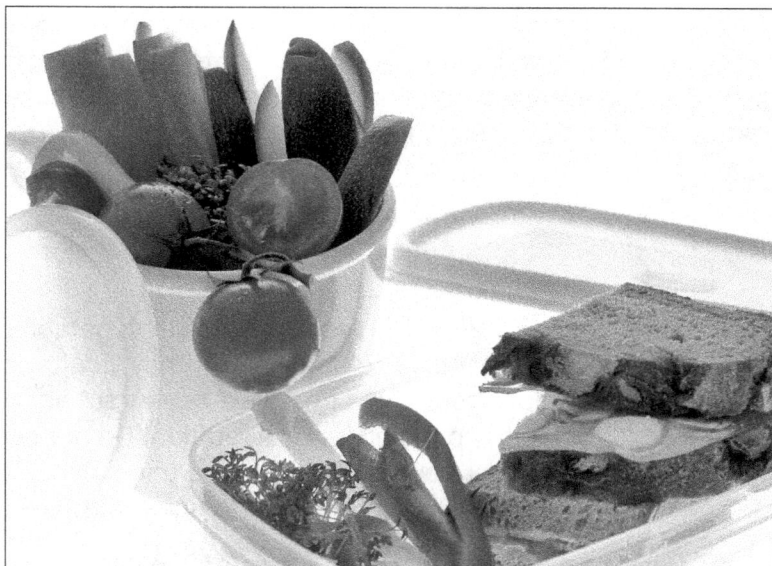

Chapter 16
Food Rotation at Work

Fuel your mind

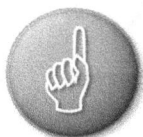

The work place does not always provide good cooking facilities and some do not even provide heating up facilities.

Bring your food in with you, lots of the dishes in the recipe section are designed to be eaten cold and lots of the hot ones taste great cold.

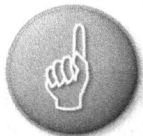

Internal meetings often take place over lunchtime and are sandwich based.

Take your own food to the meeting, even if it is only several pieces of fruit. Or ask the meeting planner to get you some fruit. You can always eat something else at your desk either before or after the meeting if you are still hungry.

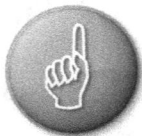

External meetings often happen in restaurants.

Most restaurants will serve a piece of fish and vegetables or a piece of chicken and vegetables and if they don't, do your best. The golden rule is: Do not see a restaurant as an excuse to abandon the principles of the rotation. Do not eat thick creamy sauces or have a plate of extra thick chips or decide to have a double chocolate cake to finish with.

Restaurant food can and will fit into the rotation if you think before you order.

Adapting the rotation plan for work

It is really easy to adapt any rotation for work. If we take the first, very limited, rotation and use it in a situation where there are no cooking or heating up facilities it would not take much modification, in fact only the lunch meal would need to be changed each day.

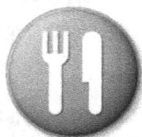

Day 1 Swap the lunch recipe of Plaice for a mixed bean salad (see recipe)

Day 2 Take the Lemon and Lime Prawns with you in a tupperware and the lettuce and herb salad separately and combine the two at your desk.

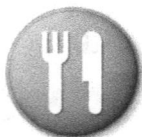

Day 3 Replace grilled cod with vegetarian carrot and coriander soup. Either take the hot soup with you in a flask or have it cold which is equally delicious.

Day 4 Bake the potato the night before or in the morning and take a tin of tuna in brine with you. Eat this accompanied with batons of raw cucumber.

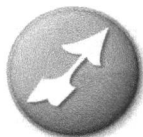

Tips for eating at work

All fruit and vegetables can be taken to work either in their raw or a cooked state these can easily be eaten at your desk or in a parked car between meetings.

All nuts can be taken to work and again eaten in the office or even in the corridor between meetings.

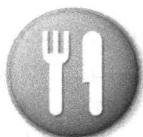

Dishes like Quick Turkey (see recipe) can be eaten as a snack with your fingers in a parked car or at your desk.

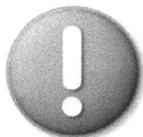

I found that sometimes I would run the rotation from evening to evening, as opposed to from breakfast to breakfast. I would cook a double portion of the evening meal and then have the second half for lunch the next day. Ok it means you eat the same meal twice, but how often do you do that anyway? You would not think it unusual to have roast chicken at night and chicken salad for lunch the next day would you? And what about all those weeks where you ate the same sandwich for lunch Monday to Friday?

All the recipes deliberately limit the number of families used at any one time so that you can create a week with the maximum variety. If there is an item in a family, and you do not want to eat that family on that day, either because you want to save it for another day or do not like it, then just omit the item.

All the recipes are designed to be extremely quick to produce so that you can create them even when you are feeling tired after a long day at work. They are mostly a generous portion for 1 person, with the exception of the whole chicken dishes and some of the stews, so if you are cooking for your family just multiply the ingredients accordingly.

When you get started on this plan you will find that the recipes for dishes are literally endless. I have offered a selection in each category in Chapters 17 and 18 so that the principles of the rotation and how to mix your foods become clear. All of the recipes can be adapted for you to add the particular foods that you like and omit some of my suggestions if they do not agree with you or you do not like the taste of that particular food.

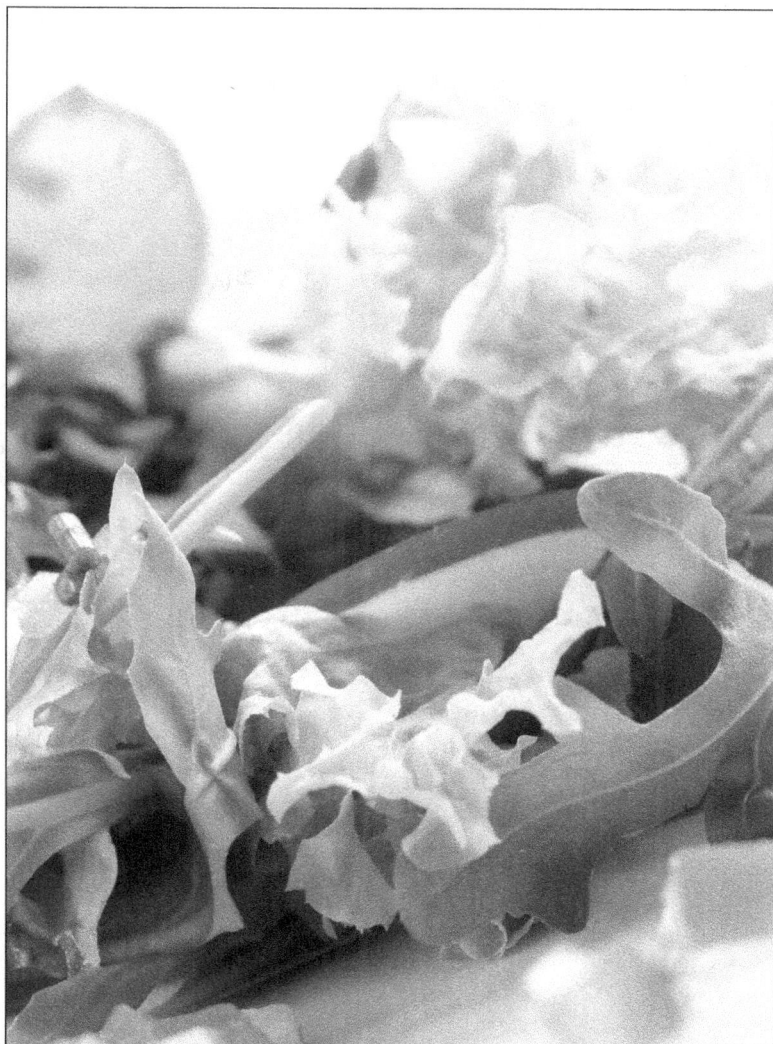

Chapter 17
Recipes for the Working Day

Recipes for Shellfish

Lemon and Lime Prawns

Ingredients

Large portion of prawns peeled cooked
2 Lemons
1 Lime
Chopped dill
Salt
Pepper

Method

Put peeled prawns into a large bowl and squeeze juice of 2 lemons and one lime over them, add roughly chopped dill and salt and pepper to taste

Eat with rice cakes or corn cakes Family Rice

Families:
Crustacean;
Citrus

Recipes for Shellfish

Prawn Cocktail no Mayonnaise

Ingredients

4oz 113gms peeled cooked prawns
2 lemons
1 spring onion chopped very finely
Several sprigs of flat parsley
Several sprigs of fresh basil
Iceberg lettuce
Salt and Pepper

Method

Put the peeled prawns in a bowl and cover with lemon juice

Add the finely chopped onion and half the parsley chopped, mix together well and add black pepper and a little salt.

Roughly shred the lettuce and add torn basil leaves and torn parsley leaves

Pile the prawns on top of the lettuce and serve. Take the lettuce to work wrapped separately to keep it fresh

Families:
Crustacean; Citrus;
Lily; Sunflower

Recipes for Shellfish

Avocado and Prawns with Lemon Juice

Ingredients

1 x large avocado
4oz 113gms frozen cooked peeled prawns
1 x lemon

Method

Halve the avocado and remove stone, squeeze lemon juice over both halves

Defrost prawns and drain well. Drench prawns in lemon juice and add pepper to taste

Spoon into avocado halves and serve

Take the avocado to work separately and combine with prawns just before serving. If you need to prepare the avocado in advance use lots of lemon juice because this will stop it discolouring

Families:
Crustacean; Avocado;
Citrus

Recipes for Fish

Tuna Fish with Cucumber

Ingredients

Tuna Fish
Cucumber
Rice Cakes
Preferably use fresh cooked Tuna but tinned would do if really necessary

Method

Flake fish and add salt and pepper and herbs (basil or tarragon) to taste
Slice a third of a cucumber off
Cut off most of skin and slice in two lengthwise
Scoop out soft flesh and mix with tuna fish
Slice remaining cucumber to use as garnish
Pile tuna and cucumber mixture on rice cakes and garnish with remaining slices, serve
Take the rice cakes to work wrapped separately to keep them crisp

Families:
Mackerel; Gourd;
Grass

Recipes for Chicken & Turkey

Quick Turkey

Ingredients

As much turkey as you like

Fresh herbs

Method

Dampen the base of a thin pan with olive oil from a mista and add turkey and fresh herbs - suggest basil or tarragon or thyme - whatever you like. Fry for 8 - 10 minutes turning often. Leave to cool and take to work in foil or Tupperware

Eat this with your raw vegetables of the day, carrot batons work well. Family Carrot

Families:
Turkey

Recipes for Chicken & Turkey

Quick Chilli Turkey or Chicken

Ingredients

As much turkey or chicken as you like
Fresh herbs
Fresh chilli chopped really small

Method

Dampen the base of a thin pan with olive oil and add turkey or chicken and chilli. Fry for 8 - 10 minutes turning often

When nearly cooked add fresh herbs to taste - coriander works well, leave to cool and take to work in foil or Tupperware

Eat this with your raw vegetables of the day, or a salad

Families:
Turkey Or Pheasant;
Potato

Recipes for Chicken & Turkey

Cold Turkey or Chicken

Ingredients

As much cold, roasted turkey or chicken as you like

Fresh herbs

Method

Cut the cold turkey or chicken into chunks and mix with shredded lettuce, scatter with fresh herbs to taste - coriander works well, take to work in foil or Tupperware.

Eat this with your raw vegetables of the day, or salad ingredients

Families:
Turkey Or Pheasant;
Sunflower

Recipes for Chicken & Turkey

Eggs with Corn Cakes

Ingredients

Hard boiled Eggs
Fresh herbs
Corn Cakes

Method

Boil the eggs until just hard. Chop herbs, coriander works well so does parsley or dill or tarragon.

Take eggs and herbs and corn cakes to work wrapped separately.
Shell eggs slice and scatter with herbs or mash with chopped herbs and spoon onto corn cakes

Families:
Pheasant;
Grass

Recipes for Soup

Vegetarian Carrot and Coriander Soup

Ingredients

1lb 450gms carrots
Pinch of salt, pepper
1 dessertspoon coriander seeds
Sprigs of fresh coriander
1pt 600ml vegetable stock
(can use cube if essential)

Method

Scrub and slice carrots and bring to boil in stock
Add coriander seeds
Add generous sprigs of fresh coriander
Simmer for 15 - 20 minutes
Liquidise soup and either re heat and put in flask or
Leave to cool
Serve sprinkled with fresh coriander

Families:
Carrot

Recipes for Jacket Potato

Jacket Potato

All of the jacket potato recipes in Chapter 18 would work with a cold baked potato see pages 197- 201

Families:
As per recipe

Recipes for Salad

Cauliflower and Coriander Salad

Ingredients

- 1 cauliflower
- Juice of 1 lemon
- 1tbs 5ml coriander seeds
- Salt and pepper
- Fresh coriander

Method

Wash the cauliflower and divide into small florets
Mix lemon juice and coriander seeds together with
salt and pepper
Toss cauliflower in dressing and then spray with olive
oil and re toss
Sprinkle with chopped fresh coriander

Families:
Mustard;
Carrot

Recipes for Salad

Melon Salad

Ingredients

A quarter of a melon
Salt and pepper
Paprika
Juice of half a lemon
1 bunch watercress
Quarter of a cucumber

Method

Cut melon from skin and cut into small pieces
Mix salt pepper and lemon juice with a pinch of paprika
Pour over melon and cover
Leave to stand for an hour
Roughly chop the watercress and mix with melon
Skin and chop the cucumber and garnish the dish

Families:
Gourd; Citrus;
Mustard

Recipes for
Salad

Tuna Salad in Grapefruit

Ingredients

1 grapefruit
Fresh cooked tuna (tinned in brine if absolutely
necessary)
Lettuce
Chick peas

Method

Cut grapefruit in half
Cut out flesh and section it removing all pulp
Line shell with shredded lettuce and squeeze juice of
grapefruit back into shell
Mix grapefruit pulp and chickpeas to taste and add
flaked tuna
Heap mixture back into shells and sprinkle with
paprika
Serve

Families:
Citrus; Mackerel;
Sunflower; Pea

Recipes for Salad

Lettuce and Herb Salad

Ingredients

Half an Iceburg lettuce
Fresh Coriander, Mint and Basil

Method

Roughly chop lettuce or pull apart with fingers
Chop herbs or pull apart with fingers

Sprinkle herbs onto lettuce and toss to mix well
Serve

Families:
Sunflower

Recipes for Salad

Banana Raisin and Carrot Salad

This recipe is good if you need something sweet as a snack or accompaniment to meat or fish

Ingredients

2 bananas
1oz 28 gms raisins
1oz 28 gms almonds roughly chopped
1 large carrot grated finely

Method

Slice bananas thinly and mix with raisins and rough chopped almonds and grated carrot

Serve in bowl garnished with parsley

Families:
Banana; Grape;
Prunus Rose

Recipes for Salad

Stuffed Apple Salad

Ingredients

1 apple
2 lettuce leaves shredded
Brazil nuts chopped or other nut if you prefer
but not peanuts
1 banana chopped
Cress

Method

Wash apple and core
Scoop out flesh with teaspoon and chop
Mix shredded lettuce with nuts banana and apple flesh
Fill apple with mixture and garnish with cress

Families:
Pome Rose; Sunflower;
Brazil; Banana; Mustard

Recipes for Salad

Mixed Bean Salad

Ingredients

1 Portion Kidney Beans
1 Portion Cannellini Beans
1 Portion Chick Peas
1 Portion Butter Beans

Method

For this recipe for work you might find
it easier to use tinned beans.
Drain water from beans and chick peas
Mix all the ingredients together and add herbs of
choice
Add squeeze of lemon juice, salt and pepper
Serve

Families:
Pea

Recipes for Fruit Dishes

Bananas and Brazil Nuts

Ingredients

2 Bananas
Handful of Brazil Nuts

Method

Eat them whole together or mash the bananas and add chopped Brazil nuts to the top

Families:
Banana;
Brazil

Recipes for Fruit Dishes

Exotic Fruit Salad

Ingredients

- 1 Banana
- 1 Nectarine
- 2 Apricots
- 3 Plums

Method

Peel the banana and roughly chop, slice nectarine, apricots and plums and combine together. If not eating immediately, add a squeeze of lemon juice to prevent the fruit from discolouring

Families:
Banana;
Prunus Rose

Recipes for Fruit Dishes

Mixed Citrus Bowl

Ingredients

- 1 Orange
- 1 Pink Grapefruit
- 2 Clementines or Mandarins

Method

Peel, de pith and chop all the fruit
Combine together in a bowl

Families:
Citrus

Recipes for
Fruit Dishes

Kiwi and Strawberries

Ingredients

2 kiwi
12 Strawberries

Method

Halve the kiwi and scoop the flesh out with a spoon
Roughly chop the kiwi flesh
Hull and chop the strawberries
Combine together in a bowl

Families:
Actinidia;
Berry Rose

Recipes for
Fruit Dishes

Melon Cocktail

Ingredients

2 generous slices of watermelon
2 generous slices of honeydew melon

Method

Roughly chop the melon flesh or use a melon baller
Combine together in a bowl

Families:
Gourd

Recipes for Fruit Dishes

Oat Bran with Orange Juice

Ingredients

   1 Portion of Oat Bran
   Orange Juice to taste
   1 Orange peeled and de pithed

Method

Put the oat bran in a bowl and pour orange juice over
to taste
Slice orange and scatter on top
Serve

Families:
Grass;
Citrus

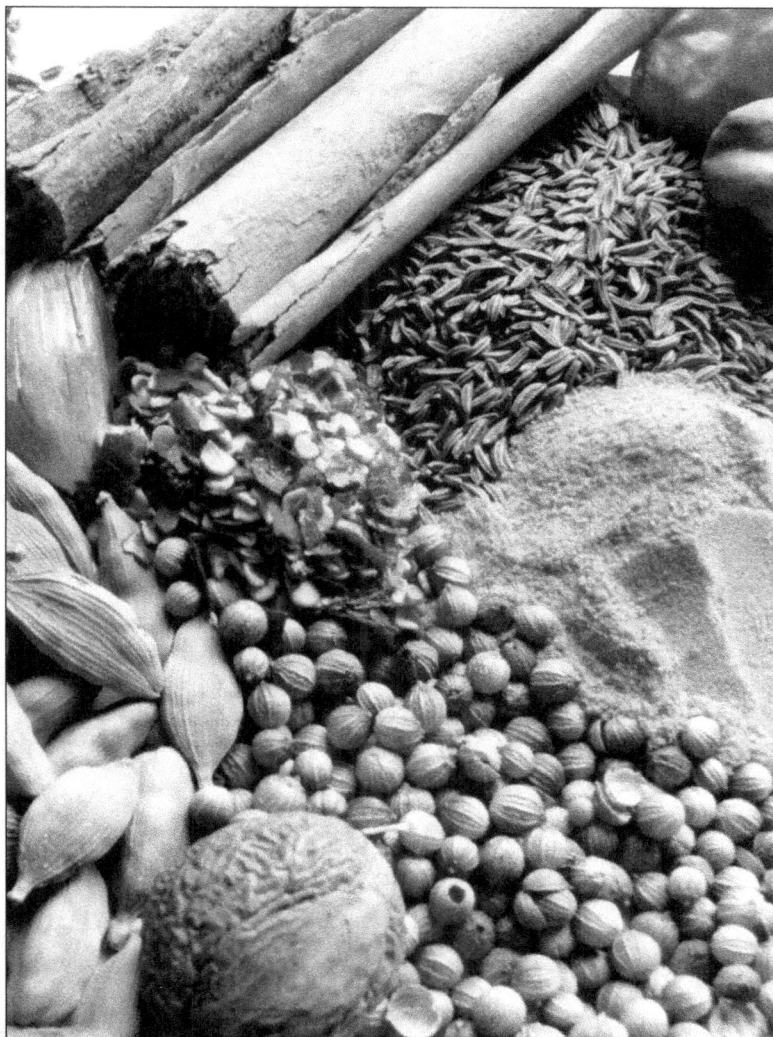

Chapter 18
Meals More Easily Eaten at Home

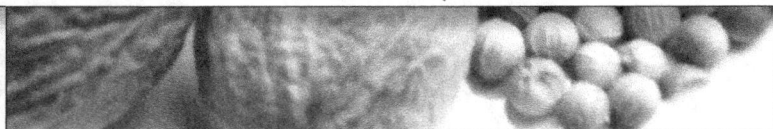

Recipes for Fish & Chicken

Tasty Parcels

This is a really versatile idea and can be made with Chicken or if you prefer Fish. Try it with Salmon or Trout

Ingredients

1 Salmon Steak or one whole trout gutted and cleaned or one cooked chicken breast
Splash Water
Scraping vegetable spread
Sprigs of fresh tarragon to taste
Salt & Freshly Ground Black Pepper

Method

Place the fish or chicken in the middle of a square of tin foil and add the splash of water, scraping of vegetable spread, tarragon, salt and pepper.

Fold tin foil loosely around the fish or Chicken and put in a pre heated oven 375F/190C Gas mark 5 for 25 minutes for the fish or chicken

It can also be made with a cooked cold chicken breast instead of the fish. In this case reduce the cooking time to 15 minutes

Families:
Salmon or Pheasant

Recipes for Fish & Chicken

Tasty Cod Parcels

This is a small variation on the above which can be made with any member of the Cod family

Ingredients

1 fish steak
Splash grape juice
Scraping vegetable spread
Handful of green or red grapes, halved and pitted
Sprigs of fresh tarragon
Salt & freshly ground black pepper

Method

Place the fish in the middle of a square of tin foil and add a handful of pitted and halved grapes, the splash of grape juice, scraping of vegetable spread, tarragon, salt and pepper

Fold tin foil loosely around the fish and put in a pre heated oven 375F/190C Gas mark 5 for 25 minutes

Families:
Cod;
Grape

Recipes for Fish & Chicken

Cod or Chicken with Mediterranean Topping

Ingredients

> 1 fillet of cod
> 1 onion
> Green and red (bell) pepper chopped – use half
> or the whole depending on taste
> 8oz (225g) tomatoes skinned and chopped
> Fresh Marjoram chopped

Method

Lightly sauté the chopped onion and peppers then stir
in the chopped tomatoes and simmer for a couple of
minutes

Chop the fish into cubes and carefully add to the
vegetable mixture

Simmer for 20 minutes and serve

Alternatively roast cod in the oven and top with the
sautéed vegetables as above

This recipe also works
with Haddock

Families:
Cod or Pheasant;
Lily; Potato

Recipes for
Fish & Chicken

Rice with Fish and Chicken

This can be made with any chunky fish and chicken
and shellfish. Below is a suggestion

Ingredients

4oz 113gms fresh chicken cubed
4oz 113 gms cod
6oz 170gms fresh prawns in shells
4oz 113gms fresh artichoke hearts
3 tomatoes
1 green pimento
2 cloves of garlic
8oz 226 gms Arborio rice
Pinch of saffron

Families:
Pheasant; Cod; Crustacean;
Sunflower; Potato

Method

Put a mist of oil in a heavy bottomed pan and fry
chicken and fish and prawns. Add rice and a little
water and stir until rice has absorbed water. Continue to
add water a little at a time. Add prepared artichoke
hearts and thinly sliced pimento and chopped
tomatoes. Continue adding water stirring continuously until
rice is soft. Serve immediately

If you have some food left over, freeze it with a label
it for your next rotation

Recipes for Fish

Fish kebabs

This is another versatile recipe – use the ideas below as a guideline – any chunky fish that will stay on a kebab skewer will do

Ingredients

150g/5oz monkfish
150g/5oz Salmon steak
Large prawns uncooked

Method

Cut the monkfish and salmon into cubes and shell the prawns

Thread them onto a metal skewer and grill kebabs to seal them

Place in a hot oven 425f 220c gas mark 7 to cook for 4 – 5 minutes

Families:
Angler; Salmon

Recipes for Fish

There are many dishes that can be done in the microwave if that style of cooking does not affect you. If it does, replace the microwave with a traditional steamer

Microwave Steamed Fish

Ingredients

  1 fillet of plaice
  1 teaspoon peeled and finely grated root ginger
  2 spring onions finely chopped

Method

Place the fish in the microwave steamer with a little water under the plate
Steam for 2 minutes
Add ginger and steam for 1 minute
Add onions and steam for a further minute
Serve
Note timings may vary with different microwaves

Families:
Plaice; Lily; Ginger

Recipes for Fish

Tuna kebabs and Baked Aubergine

Ingredients

- 1 fresh tuna steak
- 7oz 200g small mushrooms
- 1lb 450g tomatoes
- 6 garlic cloves
- 4 aubergines

Families:
Mackerel; Fungi;
Potato

Method

Wash mushrooms and trim stalks cut them in half.
Cut tuna into cubes. Skin and seed tomatoes and cut
the flesh of 2 into pieces like the mushrooms
Peel and finely chop the shallot. Sweat the cut
tomatoes cook for 10 mins
Blanch the unpeeled garlic in hot water for 5 minutes
and drain. Cut aubergines lengthwise and brush with
oil. Bake aubergine in oven on top of garlic
Thread tuna mushrooms and tomato onto skewers and
brush with oil. Grill until cooked
Take aubergine and garlic from oven and crush the
cloves adding crushed clove to diced tomatoes
Coat the aubergine halves with tomato and garlic
mixture and top with tuna kebabs

Recipes for Fish

Sea Bass or Trout with Almonds and Orange

Ingredients

Families:
Bass or Salmon;
Citrus; Rose Stone

1 trout or 1 sea bass
Scraping of vegetable spread
Juice of 1 orange
Flaked Almonds
Orange segments for garnish

Method

Pat the fish dry and brush the inside with orange juice

Scatter the flaked almonds over the fish, turn and scatter over the other side

Bake in oven dish for 14 minutes turning once 450F 230C gas mark 8

Note this dish tastes good with lemon juice instead of orange juice if desired

Recipes for Fish

Plaice with Prawns

Ingredients

1 fillet of plaice
Mist of olive oil
2 shallots finely chopped
1 tablespoon of peeled cooked prawns
Fresh parsley
Large splash of mineral water

Method

Cut the plaice in two lengthwise
Sauté the shallots until soft and add prawns and parsley. Spoon mixture into the two plaice fillets
Roll these securing them with a cocktail stick
Put plaice in oven proof dish and add large splash of water
Cover with foil and bake 400F 200C gas mark 6 for 20 minutes

Families:
Plaice; Crustacean;
Lily

Recipes for Fish

Mackerel with Courgettes

Ingredients

> Fresh Mackerel
> Courgettes

Method

Grill the mackerel with a little salt and pepper 5 minutes per side

Slice the courgettes into chunks and boil in salted water for 3 minutes

Drain courgettes and serve generous quantities with grilled mackerel

Families:
Mackerel;
Gourd

Recipes for Fish

Grilled Cod

Ingredients

Cod

Method

Grill the cod with a little salt and pepper 5 - 8 minutes per side depending on thickness

Squeeze lemon over to serve

Families:
Cod

Recipes for Fish

Grilled Haddock

Ingredients

Haddock

Method

Grill the Haddock with a little salt and pepper 5 - 8 minutes per side depending on thickness

Squeeze lemon over to serve

Families:
Cod

Recipes for Fish

Cod Stir-fry with Spring Onions and Leeks

Ingredients

1oz 226gms cod
1 large bunch spring onions
2 leeks

Method

Cube the cod

Finely chop leeks and onions

Put a mist of oil over base of thin bottomed frying pan or wok

Add leeks and onions and fry until soft

Add cod and continue frying stirring frequently for 3 - 5 mins

Serve

Families:
Cod;
Lily

Recipes for Fish

Grilled Plaice with Rosemary and Garlic

Ingredients

1 plaice
Fresh rosemary 3 sprigs
1 clove fresh garlic

Method

Put fish into grill pan

Add half the rosemary sprigs and crushed fresh garlic

Grill for 5 minutes

Turn fish and add more rosemary and crushed garlic to other side

Grill for further 5 minutes and serve

Families:
Plaice

Recipes for Fish

Scampi Provencal

Ingredients

8oz 226gms fresh or frozen scampi
1 onion
2 tomatoes
3 large mushrooms
1 clove garlic

Families:
Crustacean; Lily;
Potato; Fungi

Method

Defrost scampi if necessary
In a thin based pan with a mist of oil or scraping of
margarine fry thinly sliced onion and garlic together
until soft
Skin and slice tomatoes and mushrooms and add to
onion
Mix well and add scampi
Fry for approximately 3 - 5 minutes
Garnish with parsley and lemon juice
If desired, serve with rice

Recipes for
Fish

Monkfish with Rice and Red Peppers

Ingredients

6oz 170gms monkfish
Rice
Red peppers

Method

Cube monkfish into chunks
Add to microwave steamer with some water
Steam for 3 - 4 minutes on full power
Boil rice with bay leaf and herbs to taste
Dice peppers and soften in thick bottomed pan with a
scraping of spread
When rice is soft add to pan and mix well
Add monkfish and heat through for a couple of
minutes.
Serve

Families:
Angler; Grass;
Potato

Recipes for Fish

Sea Bass with Asparagus and Onions

Ingredients

1 sea bass whole - gutted and cleaned
Asparagus to taste
1 large onion

Method

Add seasoning to fish and steam whole sea bass in microwave steamer with water in base for 7 minutes or until nearly cooked

Dice onion and cut asparagus into chunks

Add to steamer and finish cooking for approximately 3 - 4 minutes on high

Serve

Families:
Bass;
Lily

Recipes for Fish

Fish Cakes

These can be made with cod, or any firm white fish, salmon, prawn or crab

Ingredients

> Cooked fish of your choice
> 2 large potatoes
> Herbs of choice

Method

Peel potatoes slice and bring to the boil in salted water. Boil until soft - 10 minutes.
Mash potato with herbs of choice and a scraping of spread. Take cooked fish and flake into potato mash.
Mix well, add a little paprika and salt and pepper to taste
Form mixture into patties and place on baking tray in preheated oven 180 degrees F 80 degrees C and bake for approximately 15 minutes

Serve

Families:
Fish as per family;
Potato

Recipes for Fish

Trout with Mint and Orange

Ingredients

- 1 x whole trout - gutted and cleaned
- 2 x oranges
- Fresh mint

Method

Slice 1 orange in half and squeeze out juice and as much pulp as possible.

Fill fish cavity with orange pulp and fresh mint leaves

Place fish in microwave steamer and fill base with water.

Pour orange juice over fish and steam on full power for 5 - 6 minutes.

Peel and de pith second orange and cut into thin slices.

Use orange slices to garnish cooked fish to taste.

Families:
Salmon;
Citrus

Recipes for Fish

Poached salmon with Lettuce Peas and Onions

Families:
Salmon; Sunflower;
Pea; Lily

Ingredients

- 1 x salmon fillet
- Quarter of an iceberg lettuce
- Frozen peas to taste
- 1 small onion

Method

Place clean salmon fillet in microwave steamer with water in the base. Season with salt and pepper and basil.

Cook for 5 minutes on high

Slice lettuce into chunks

Slice onion very thinly

Add lettuce and onion to peas in a small pan and just cover with water. Add basil and salt and pepper.

Bring to boil and simmer for approximately 1 minute

Drain and serve with poached salmon.

Garnish with fresh basil if desired

Serve

Recipes for Fish

Mixed Grilled Fish with Lemon

This dish can be made with all firm fish and the ingredients below are a suggestion of a good mixture but are not exhaustive

Ingredients

    4oz 113 gms fresh salmon fillet (organic if possible)
    4oz 113 gms fresh cod
    4oz 113 gms fresh haddock
    4oz 113 gms fresh octopus
    2 large prawns peeled

Method

Cut all the fish and octopus into chunks, leave the prawns whole. Scatter fish in grill pan and squeeze juice of one lemon over top.
Add salt, pepper and herbs to taste - try fresh dill and fresh basil. Cook fish on high turning occasionally for approximately 10 minutes

Serve

Families:
Salmon; Cod; Plaice;
Mollusc; Crustacean

Recipes for
Fish

Sole with Prawns

Ingredients

8oz 226gms fresh sole
4oz 113 gms cooked prawns

Method

Heat grill, cut the fish into two portions
Grill the sole with a little salt and pepper for 5
minutes on each side
Heap the prawns into the grill pan and heat through
at the end of the cooking time
When ready to serve put first piece of fish on plate
and cover with prawns
Sprinkle with lemon juice and fresh herbs to taste
Place second piece of sole on top and sprinkle with
lemon juice and fresh herbs to taste

Families:
Sole;
Crustacean

Recipes for Fish

Trout and Salad

Ingredients

Trout
Lettuce
Grated Carrot

Method

Take whole gutted trout and put in microwave steamer with water underneath.

Sprinkle with a little garlic salt

Microwave for 5 - 6 minutes

Serve with fresh salad of lettuce leaves and grated carrot with fresh coriander

Families:
Salmon; Sunflower;
Carrot

Recipes for Fish

Sardines with Tomatoes

Ingredients

2 large fresh sardines
4 large tomatoes
1 large onion

Families:
Herring; Potato;
Lily

Method

Clean sardines and grill under hot grill with a sprinkling of garlic salt for 3 - 4 minutes each side
Skin and chop tomatoes and onion.
Gently soften onion in thin bottomed pan with a mist of oil.
Add tomatoes and cook until tender - approximately 5 minutes.
Serve sardines and pour tomato and onion mixture over the top. Serve with fresh herbs of choice

This recipe also works well with Red Snapper - grill for 8 - 10 minutes Family: Snapper

Recipes for
Fish

Salmon and Cod kebabs

Ingredients

Salmon fillet cut into cubes
Half a cod fillet cut into cubes
Red and green peppers chopped in cubes

Method

Thread alternate pieces of salmon, pepper and cod onto metal skewers

Grill under hot grill turning frequently for approximately 8 - 10 minutes

Serve

Families:
Salmon; Cod;
Potato

Recipes for Fish

Salmon and rice Noodles

Ingredients

1 salmon fillet
Half a small packet of rice noodles

Method

Cook fillet in microwave dish with water in bottom for 6 - 7 minutes

Place rice noodles in boiling water for 4 - 6 minutes

Drain and add flaked salmon, mix well with a small amount of lemon juice and serve hot

Families:
Salmon;
Grass

Recipes for Fish

Chilli Fish

Ingredients

8oz 226gms cod or haddock or salmon
Fresh finely chopped chillies
8oz 226gms kidney beans
6oz 170gms fresh tomatoes skinned

Method

Soak dried kidney beans according to instructions (if desperate us a tin of kidney beans)

Put a mist of oil in a thick bottomed pan and slowly cook the cubed fish through.

Add kidney beans tomatoes and finely chopped chillies

Stir then cover and simmer for 15 minutes stirring occasionally

Serve with rice or salad

Families:
Cod or Salmon;
Potato; Pea

Recipes for
Shellfish

Brochette of Scallops

Ingredients

4 large scallops
Slices of fresh pineapple

Method

Wash scallops and cut in half and thread onto skewers alternating with slices of fresh pineapple

Grill under medium heat for 8 - 10 minutes turning once

Serve with rice if desired

Families:
Mollusc;
Pineapple

Recipes for Shellfish

Mussels

Ingredients

1lb 450gms mussels
1 shallot finely chopped
5 - 6 stalks parsley
1 bay leaf
Sprig of thyme
Salt and pepper
Half a pint (quarter of a litre) of water

Method

Put all ingredients into large pan and steam the mussels for approximately 10 - 15 minutes over a medium heat

Serve sprinkled with chopped parsley

Note only eat the mussels that have fully opened

Families:
Mollusc; Lily;

Recipes for Chicken & Turkey

Chicken with Asparagus

Try this with chicken or turkey for a quick and easy lunch or supper - serve with rice or potatoes depending on rotation

Ingredients

> 10oz 300g of chicken or turkey
> 2 onions
> 10 Fresh Asparagus tips

Method

Cut the meat into cubes and slice the onion into chunks.
Thread onto metal skewer alternating meat onion and asparagus.
Put under a hot grill
Grill for 12 minutes turning occasionally until chicken or turkey is thoroughly cooked

Families:
Pheasant or Turkey;
Lily

Recipes for Chicken & Turkey

Chilli Chicken

Ingredients

- 10oz 283g fresh organic chicken breasts
- Very finely chopped chillies
- Spinach
- Broccoli
- Cauliflower

Families:
Pheasant; Potato;
Beet; Mustard

Method

Cube the chicken breast

Wash spinach

Cut broccoli and cauliflower into florets

Place cubed chicken in thin-based frying pan or wok and add a mist of oil. Fry briskly adding finely chopped chillies when sealed

When nearly cooked add broccoli and cauliflower florets

Fry for further 3 - 5 minutes

Pour boiling water over spinach to wilt and bring to boil

Serve immediately

Recipes for Chicken & Turkey

Stir Fried Turkey

This makes a great fast lunch or a bigger portion for a substantial dinner

Ingredients

As much turkey as you like cut into cubes
Shredded white cabbage
Garlic Salt
Pepper

Families:

Turkey; Mustard

Method

Fry the turkey in a thin based pan in the tiniest amount of olive oil - use a spray can to just dampen the pan.
After a couple of minutes add the shredded cabbage.
Give a liberal sprinkling of garlic salt and pepper to taste
Total cooking time approximately 8 - 10 minutes stirring continuously
For a more substantial meal add cauliflower and broccoli florets at the same time as the cabbage
- they are both in the Mustard Family

Recipes for Chicken & Turkey

Roast Chicken with Lemon and Tarragon

Families:
Pheasant

Ingredients

1 whole chicken no giblets
3 Lemons
1 bunch fresh tarragon

Method

Cut the lemons into quarters and squeeze the juice over the bird then put into the cavity

Roughly cut the tarragon and place inside the cavity and on top of the bird. Cover with tin foil and place in a pre heated oven 375F/190C Gas mark 5 for 1 and a half hours or until the juices of the bird run clear

Baste frequently during cooking and remove the tin foil for the last 30 minutes of cooking to brown the skin

Serve sprinkled with chopped tarragon and with vegetables or salad of choice

Note this also works with Turkey but increase the cooking time depending on the size of the bird. Both meats can be sliced and taken to the office for lunch

Recipes for
Chicken & Turkey

Chicken on a Bed of Onions

Ingredients

1 whole chicken jointed or 4 chicken joints
4 - 5 cooking onions

Method

Roughly chop 4 - 5 onions and place in large oven proof dish.
Place chicken joints on top of onions and sprinkle with mixed herbs. Roast in a pre heated medium oven 375F/190C Gas mark 5 until chicken is cooked - approximately 45 minutes
Note by leaving the skin on the chicken the natural fat helps to baste the onions so they remain moist but still crisp nicely.
Serve with boiled leeks and asparagus if desired.
Family: lily
Freeze any left over food with a label on it and use it for a later rotation

This dish also works well and is more substantial on a bed of mixed beans, try cannellini and kidney.
Family: Pea

Families:
Pheasant; Lily

Recipes for Chicken & Turkey

Mediterranean Chicken Casserole

Ingredients

- 4 chicken joints - skin removed
- 3 cooking onions chopped
- 6 fresh plum tomatoes chopped
- 2 red peppers chopped
- Basil

Families:
Pheasant; Lily;
Potato

Method

Brown the chicken in a spray of oil

Add onions and fry till soft turning often to prevent sticking

Add red peppers and fry for further 2 minutes

Add chopped tomatoes and basil

Put in oven 375F/190C Gas mark 5 for 1- 2 hours

Serve with baked potatoes Family: Potato

Freeze any left over food with a label on it and use in your next rotation

Recipes for Vegetable Dishes

Ratatouille

Make this recipe without onions and garlic if you do not want to eat the Lily Family

Ingredients

    1 red onion
    1 cooking onion
    1 garlic clove crushed
    3 courgettes
    5 tomatoes
    1 medium aubergine

Method

Roughly chop all the vegetables and spray with a small amount of olive oil from a mista
Put in the oven 374F 190C Gas mark 5 for 20 - 25 minutes stirring occasionally

Families:

Lily; Gourd;
Potato

Recipes for Vegetable Dishes

Lily Family Ratatouille

Ingredients

- Asparagus
- Leeks
- Onions
- Garlic

Method

Roughly chop all the vegetables and spray with a small amount of olive oil from a mista

Put in the oven 374F 190C Gas mark 5 for 20 – 25 minutes stirring occasionally

Families:
Lily

Recipes for Vegetable Dishes

Ratatouille Bake

Ingredients

    1 aubergine
    3 courgettes
    6 tomatoes

Method

Peel the aubergine and wash and trim the courgettes slice all the vegetables

Spay the bottom of an oven dish with either vegetable or olive oil and layer vegetables as follows

Tomatoes, courgette, tomatoes aubergine

Put in the oven 374F 190C Gas mark 5 for 20 - 25 minutes

Families:

Potato; Gourd;

Recipes for Vegetable Dishes

Vegetable Kebabs

Ingredients

Peppers red green and yellow
Aubergine
Tomatoes
Onions
Mushrooms (leave out if suffer from Candida)

Method

Roughly chop all the vegetables and thread onto wooden or metal skewers

Spray with olive oil and grill for 10 - 15 minutes turning occasionally

Families:
Potato; Lily;
Fungi

Recipes for Vegetable Dishes

Winter Warmer

Ingredients

- 1 Swede
- 1 turnip
- 2 carrots
- 1 leek
- Bouquet Garni

Method

Roughly cut all the vegetables put in casserole dish and pour over half a pint of boiling vegetable stock

Add bouquet garni and put in oven 375F 180C Gas Mark 4 for an hour

Families:

Mustard; Carrot; Lily

Recipes for Vegetable Dishes

Carrot and Parsnip Mash

Ingredients

3 Carrots
2 Parsnips

Method

Roughly cut the vegetables put in casserole dish and pour over half a pint of boiling vegetable stock

Simmer for 10 - 15 minutes until vegetables are soft and stock is reduced

Pour off any excess stock and mash the vegetables with pepper to taste

Families:

Carrot

Recipes for Vegetable Dishes

Roasted Courgettes

Ingredients

  3 Courgettes

Method

Slice the courgettes lengthwise and then in half again

Put a mist of oil in the bottom of a roasting tin and rub the courgettes in it

Add salt and pepper to taste

Put in the oven 374F 190C Gas mark 5 for 20 - 25 minutes turning occasionally

Families:

Goud

Recipes for
Vegetable Dishes

Roasted Peppers, Tomatoes and Mushrooms

Ingredients

1 Red pepper
1 Orange pepper
10 cherry tomatoes
10 button mushrooms

Method

Slice the peppers and halve the tomatoes and mushrooms

Put a mist of oil in the bottom of a roasting tin and rub the vegetables in it

Add a generous portion of mixed herbs to taste

Put in the oven 374F 190C Gas mark 5 for 20 - 25 minutes turning occasionally

Families:
Potato;
Fungi

Recipes for Vegetable Dishes

Potato and Red Pepper Frittata

Families:

Potato; Pheasant; Lily; Mustard

Ingredients

1 onion
8 oz 250g sliced potatoes
150ml vegetable stock
5oz 150g roasted red peppers or use pimentos in brine drained
3 eggs beaten
Black pepper
Watercress to serve

Method

Place the onion and potato in a frying pan with the stock stir then cover and cook over a medium heat 10 - 12 minutes until soft
Add peppers stir again and continue cooking boiling off any remaining liquid
When pan is nearly dry pour in beaten eggs and turn heat to low
cook for 7 - 8 minutes until base of frittata is set.
Put under hot grill for 3 - 4 minutes until all is set
Grind pepper over and serve with watercress

Recipes for Soup

The secret with all the soup recipes is NOT to use too much butter or oil when cooking the vegetables off

If possible add vegetables to seasoned water without frying at all. If you do use a scraping of butter or spray of oil, leave the soup to cool before you liquidise it and skim the fat from the pan

Following are just a couple of ideas - any vegetable combinations can be used to make a good soup

Recipes for Soup

Chicken Soup

Ingredients

1 x carcass of cooked chicken eaten as a roast
3 x carrots
2 x parsnips
2 x onions
Water
Bay leaf
Thyme
Salt and Pepper

Families:

Pheasant; Carrot;
Lily

Method

Put whole carcass into a pan of seasoned water and
boil for 30 minutes. Take all meat off bones and
discard bones and any bits of skin. Leave to cool and
skim fat from top of liquid when cold.
Slice carrot and parsnip and add to water and
chicken - add more water if necessary
Add bay leaf and other herbs and bring to boil.
Simmer for 20 minutes
Leave to cool and then liquidise
Adjust seasoning and serve hot

Recipes for Soup

Carrot and Coriander Soup

Ingredients

2 onions
Scraping of butter
1 clove garlic
Pinch of salt
1lb 450gms carrots
Pepper
1 dessertspoon coriander seeds
Sprigs of fresh coriander
1pt 600ml chicken stock (can use cube if essential)

Families:

Lily; Carrot;
Pheasant

Method

Peel and slice onions and gently fry in scraping of
butter
Add crushed garlic and salt and pepper
Scrub and slice carrots and add to pan
Add coriander seeds
Add chicken stock and simmer for 15 – 20 minutes
Allow to cool and skim
Liquidise soup and re heat and adjust seasoning
Serve sprinkled with fresh coriander

Recipes for Soup

Chunky Fish Soup
- More Like a Stew

Ingredients

A Spray of oil
1 clove garlic
1 tsp ground cumin
Pinch of paprika
8oz 200g chopped tomatoes
1 red pepper
1lb 400g white fish fillets eg Cod
Handful of coriander
Lemon to garnish

Families:

Cod;
Potato

Method

Heat oil in pan. Crush garlic and add to pan with cumin and paprika. Add 4 fl oz, 100 ml water and chopped tomatoes and bring to boil. Turn down heat and add chopped and deseeded pepper. Simmer for 5 minutes
Add fish simmer for 5 minutes
Serve with coriander and a wedge of lemon

This recipe can also be made with Chicken and halved small potatoes can be added with the tomatoes if desired

Recipes for Soup

Mushroom Soup

Ingredients

1 large onion finely chopped
1 green pepper finely chopped
1 clove garlic crushed
4oz 113gms mushrooms chopped
1 pt 600ml chicken stock (can use cube if desperate)

Method
Fry onions and green pepper in scraping of butter with crushed garlic
Add mushrooms and soften
Add salt and pepper to taste
Add chicken stock and simmer for 15 - 20 minutes
Cool and skim
Liquidise
Re heat, adjust seasoning and serve with fresh parsley leaves

Families:

Fungi; Lily; Pheasant

Simple Potato Family Recipes

Jacket potatoes with a variety of fillings

For all recipes take one large potato and clean thoroughly. Either bake in microwave until soft - approximately 10 - 12 minutes or partially bake in microwave and finish in oven for a crispy skin

Alternatively bake entirely in oven - approximately 1 and half hours on gas mark 4 350 degrees C 180 degrees F

Simple Potato Family Recipes

Jacket Potato with Tuna

Ingredients

Potato
Fresh tuna steak

Families:

Potato;
Mackerel

Method

Bake potato as desired

Steam fresh tuna steak in microwave dish with water in the base

Season with salt and pepper and herbs of choice

Allow approximately 5 minutes on high per steak

When both are cooked cut potato and remove a small amount of flesh

Fluff up the remaining flesh inside with a fork

Flake tuna and add it to the removed potato and mix well

Sprinkle with paprika and return to skins and serve with herb garnish

Simple Potato Family Recipes

Jacket Potato with Mackerel

Ingredients

Potato
Fresh Mackerel Fillet

Families:

Potato;
Mackerel

Method

Bake potato as desired

Steam fresh mackerel fillet in microwave dish with water in the base

Season with salt and pepper and herbs of choice

Allow approximately 5 minutes on high per steak

When both are cooked cut potato and remove a small amount of flesh

Fluff up the remaining flesh inside with a fork

Flake mackerel and add it to the removed potato and mix well

Sprinkle with paprika and return to skins and serve with herb garnish

Simple Potato Family Recipes

Jacket Potato with Prawns

Ingredients

Potato
6oz 170gms large cooked frozen prawns
Juice and pulp of 1 x lemon
Juice and pulp of 1 x orange

Method

Defrost prawns and cover with orange and lemon juice and pulp

Mix well and season with pepper

Cut potato and remove a small amount of flesh

Fluff up the remaining flesh inside with a fork

Add prawns to the removed potato and mix well

Sprinkle with paprika and return to skins and serve with herb garnish

Families:

Potato; Crustacean; Citrus

Simple Potato Family Recipes

Jacket Potato with Coleslaw and Light Mayonnaise

Ingredients

1 x large potato
2oz 57gms carrot
1 small onion chopped
1oz 28 gms sultanas
1ox 28 gms cabbage
Juice of 1 lemon
Juice of 1 orange
1 desert spoon mayonnaise

Families:

Potato; Carrot; Mustard; Lily; Grape

Method

Cook potato as above

Shred carrot cabbage and onion

Combine in a bowl with lemon and orange juice

Add sultanas and combine potato flesh with mixture

Simple Potato Family Recipes

Stuffed Tomatoes and Peppers

Ingredients

2 large tomatoes and 2 large red peppers
Fillings as below

Families:
Potato

Method

Wash the tomatoes and peppers and cut the top off
Scoop the seeds out and fill with:
* Chopped prawns and shredded lettuce
  families: Crustacean and sunflower
* Grated carrot and coriander families: carrot
* Chopped hard boiled eggs and chopped gherkins
  families: pheasant and gourd
* Boiled rice and yellow peppers families: grass and potato
* Flaked tuna fish and sweet corn families:
  mackerel and corn
* Cooked mushrooms and onions families: fungi and lily

Note this also works well when served hot to do this
soften mushrooms and onions in a heavy based pan
with a mist of oil for a couple of minutes
Pile into peppers and tomatoes and put whole into
microwave for 4 minutes on high
Or oven bake in hot oven for 20 minutes

Recipes for Salads

White Fish and Anchovy Salad

Ingredients

8oz 226gms cod or other white fish
2 tablespoons of water
1 tablespoon of lemon juice
1 bunch chopped parsley
1 bunch chopped chives
Lettuce leaves
1oz anchovy fillets if desired (note do not use many because they are processed)
black pitted olives

Families:

Cod; Citrus; Sunflower; Herring; Olive

Method

Place fish in oven proof dish and cover
Cook for 15 -20 minutes in fairly hot oven 350 degree f 180 degrees C Gas 4
Allow to cool and flake fish removing all skin and bones
Stir in the lemon juice and parsley and chives and arrange on top of shredded lettuce
Add anchovy fillets if desired and scatter black olives over

Recipes for Salads

Pea and Bean Salad

Ingredients

1 Portion of peas
1 Portion of French Beans
1 Portion of Kidney Beans

Method

Boil the peas beans and kidney beans separately until soft

Refresh with cold water

Mix all ingredients together

Add herbs to taste

Add squeeze of lemon juice, salt and pepper

Serve

Families:

Pea

Recipes for Hot Desserts

Lovely deserts can be made from any fresh fruit combined and heated in the oven. The golden rule is do not add sugar.

Baked Bananas and Nectarines

Ingredients

  1 whole banana
  1 nectarine

Method

Slice banana lengthwise

Peel and slice nectarine into batons

Place nectarine batons inside sliced banana

Wrap in foil and bake in hot oven for 20 minutes

Families:

Banana;
Prunus Rose

Recipes for Hot Desserts

Baked Apples

Ingredients

1 desert apple
2 plums

Method

Core apple and remove half of the flesh

Peel and de stone plums and chop flesh

Pile inside apple and bake in hot oven for 20 minutes

Families:

Pome rose;
Prunus rose

Recipes for Hot Desserts

Rhubarb with Orange

Ingredients

8oz 226gms Rhubarb
Zest of an Orange or peel very thinly sliced
Juice from Orange

Method

Cut wash and drain the rhubarb put in a casserole dish

Add zest or peel and mix well

Squeeze juice over and leave 24 hours

Cover casserole and put in cool oven Gas mark2 150C
or 300F for 30 minutes

Serve warm or cold

Families:

Buckwheat;
Citrus

Recipes for Cold Desserts

Raw Fruit Purée

Ingredients

    2 apricots
    Handful of raisins
    1 dessert apple cored and sliced
    Half a lemon

Method

Put apple slices in a blender with a dash of water and lemon juice

Blend until smooth

Add apricots and raisins and another squeeze of lemon and blend until smooth.

Pour into glass bows and sprinkle with Coconut if desired Family Palm

Families:

Prunus Rose; Grape;
Pome Rose; Citrus

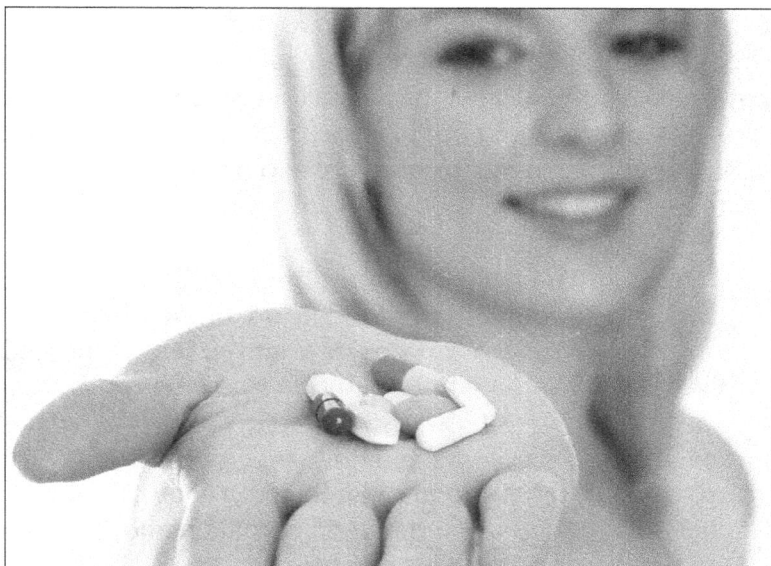

Chapter 19
Vitamins & Minerals

Vitamins and their importance to health

If you are feeling tired and run down vitamin and mineral supplements, in conjunction with a balanced diet, can really help you. It is best to take vitamin supplements along with food and also it is advisable to split the daily dose between meals.

Every person's body is different and each person will need different amounts of vitamins and minerals in order to maintain optimum health. This section is a guide as to what is available and what is known to help energy production in the body.

Every manufacturer gives a suggested daily intake and these should be followed unless your medical practitioner advises otherwise. For most vitamins the daily requirements are very low – less than 100mg but in times of stress, tiredness and lethargy you may need a higher dose to boost your immune system.

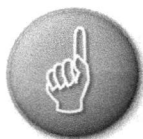

The body does not manufacture vitamins, it gets them from food or supplements. Modern processing strips most of the vitamins and minerals from the food.

In the tables below which show the food sources for vitamins, some of the foods mentioned are on the No Go list, however they are included for information and for when you are able to eat these foods again.

Understanding vitamins

Vitamins can be divided into 2 groups:

Fat soluble vitamins and **water soluble vitamins**

Fat soluble A, D, E and K

They dissolve in fat before they are absorbed in the blood stream to carry out their functions. Excesses of these vitamins are stored in the liver, because they are stored, they are not needed every day in the diet.

Water-soluble B – Complex and C

They dissolve in water and are not stored by the body, they are eliminated in urine. Therefore, we need a continuous supply of them in our diets.

Fat soluble vitamins A, D, E, K

All these are essential nutrients. Although essential, it is possible to have too much of these fat soluble vitamins. The body stores them in the gut and Vitamins A and D can be toxic at high levels.

Main sources of fat soluble vitamins

Vitamin	Role in the body	Sources
Vitamin A	Important for maintaining skin and mucous membranes, also helps with eyesight and helps the body utilise Iron properly	Apricots, Asparagus, Broccoli, Cantaloupe, Carrots, Chard, Collards, Cress, Kale, Mango, Pumpkin, Spinach, Sweet Potato, Turnip, Greens, dark green leaves, Winter Squash, Liver, Milk and Milk Products, Fish Oils, Margarine
Vitamin D	Important for healthy bones and teeth. Can also possibly help to maintain the appetite	Fish Oils, Eggs, Dairy products, Margarine

Vitamin E	Important for protecting the joints from oxidation and may also help against heart disease	Vegetable oils, leafy green vegetables, Soya Beans, Eggs
Vitamin K	Involved in blood clotting	Vegetables, Liver, Yoghurt, Lean Meat

Water soluble vitamins

Generally water soluble vitamins are not stored in the body so they are required in food on a regular basis. Most vitamins are used as part of enzyme molecules, and they are the chemical control substances of the blood.

Water-soluble vitamins are easily destroyed when you store food or washed out as you prepare it.

Vitamin B-complex

Eight of the water-soluble vitamins are known as the B-complex group:

Thiamin (vitamin B1), riboflavin (vitamin B2), niacin, pyridoxine (vitamin B6), folate, cobalamin (vitamin B12), biotin and pantothenic acid.

These vitamins function as coenzymes that help the body obtain energy from food. They also are important for normal appetite, good vision, healthy skin, a healthy nervous system and red blood cell formation. An enzyme is a protein that works like a catalyst in the body to prompt chemical changes in other substances; for example, breaking down food into energy.

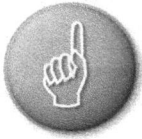

When grains and grain products are refined, much of their essential nutrients are lost. Manufacturers put nutrients back in through a process called enrichment and B-complex vitamins like thiamin, niacin, riboflavin, and folate are some of the ones frequently added along with Iron.

Examples of enriched grain products are white rice, many breakfast cereals, white flour, breads, and pasta.

The B vitamins

Important for the release of energy

As a complex, the B vitamins are essential for the proper functioning of the nervous system and are perhaps the most important nutritional factor for healthy nerve cells. The B vitamins also play a role in the conversion of carbohydrates into energy, in the metabolism of fats and protein, and in the maintenance of muscle tone in the GI tract. They are interrelated and provide wide ranging befts to skin, hair and liver but most importantly they support the nervous system.

For anyone suffering with low energy levels, B vitamins are essential and use of them will increase your energy on a day to day basis.

Vitamin	Role in the body	Sources
Thiamin (B1)	Helps utilise carbohydrates and is important for the correct function of the nervous system, heart muscles and energy release.	Pork, Whole Grains, Organic Meats, Fish, Fruits, Eggs, Milk, Raisins, Yeast, Cereals, Nuts, Oil, Green Vegetables
Riboflavin (B2)	Helps maintain healthy growth of skin and hair and is also important for energy production in the body.	Milk, Eggs, Liver, Kidney, leafy green vegetables, Yeast
Niacin B3	Helps maintain a healthy nervous system, blood circulation and is needed for the release of energy.	Meat, Poultry, Fish, Cereals, Peanuts, Milk, Yeast, Egg
Pyridoxine (B6)	Essential for the production of antibodies and red blood cells involved in the formation of adrenalin and insulin and for the production of RNA and DNA.	Wheat germ, Soybeans, Molasses, Beef, Liver, Corn , Barley, Unpolished Rice, Yeast

Cobalamin (B12)	Needed for red blood cells and maintenance of nerve tissue. They convert carbohydrates into energy. It is essential to the functioning of the nervous system and good for skin, hair and the liver	Liver, Eggs, Cheese, Milk, Fish
Pantothenic acid	Involved in energy production, and aids in formation of hormones	Liver, Kidney, Meats, Egg Yolk, Whole Grains, Legumes It is also made by intestinal bacteria
Folate (folic acid)	Aids in protein metabolism, promotes red blood cell formation, prevents birth defects of spine, and brain. It also lowers homocystein levels and thus the risk of coronary heart disease and is important for function of the Thums gland which contains the body's immune response.	Liver, Kidney, dark green leafy vegetables, Meats, Fish, Whole Grains, Fortified Grains and Cereals, Legumes, Citrus Fruits, Bananas

Biotin	Helps release energy from carbohydrates, and aids in fat synthesis.	Liver, Kidney, Egg Yolk, Milk, most fresh vegetables. It is also made by intestinal bacteria.

The B complex vitamins work with other WATER SOLUBLE VITAMINS. The most well known of which is:

Vitamin C or ascorbic acid

Vitamin C is very important for anyone suffering with a lack of energy and anyone who is feeling run down. It is vital to the immune system and also helps body cells bond together so aids in wound healing and bone and tooth formation.

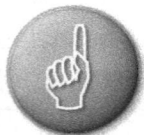

Our bodies can't make vitamin C, and they can't store large quantities of it, therefore we need to eat it every day.

Under normal conditions, if your body was optimally healthy, then eating an orange a day would give you enough vitamin C. However, if you are suffering from stress, feel tired and run down and are lacking in energy, then your body may well need considerably more. In addition if you smoke, this destroys the vitamin C in your body and you will need to take a supplement.

Antioxidants and free radicals

Vitamin C also is a powerful antioxidant. It works as a free-radical scavenger. Basically, free radicals are atoms, ions or molecules with one or more unpaired electron that bind to and destroy cellular compounds that the body needs.

An antioxidant in effect buddies up with a free electron creating an innocuous cellular compound that the body can eliminate as waste.

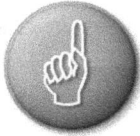

Eliminating free radicals can help improve your energy levels.

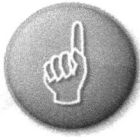

Free radicals get much of the blame for the aging process.

Vitamin	Role in the body	Sources
Ascorbic acid C	Assists in wound healing and increases resistance to infection. It is a wonderful antioxidant.	Citrus Fruits, Guava, Mango, Papaya, Strawberries, Brussels Sprouts, Green and Red Peppers, Parsley, Blackcurrants, New Potatoes, Bean Sprouts, Broccoli, Melon, Asparagus, Cabbage, Carrots, Cress, Grapes, Kale, Spinach, Tomatoes, Turnip

Minerals

The human skeleton is replaced every 7 – 10 years in adults therefore minerals that build and maintain bones are important. The main bone maintenance minerals are: Calcium, Phosphorus and Magnesium.

Mineral	Role in the body	Sources
Calcium	With phosphorus it maintains strong and healthy bones and teeth	Milk, Cheese, Yoghurt, Sesame Seeds
Phosphorus	Maintains strong bones and teeth	Milk, Fish, Meat, Poultry, Bread, Cereals
Magnesium	Maintains bones and nerve and muscle membranes. It is necessary for energy production and the metabolism of carbohydrates amino acids and fats. This vital mineral also helps utilise B-Complex vitamins, vitamin C and vitamin E	Whole Cereals, Nuts, green vegetables, Seafood, Grapefruit, Apples

Other useful minerals

Mineral	Role in the body	Sources
Iron	Used for the optimum transport of oxygen to cells which is needed for energy	Red Meat, Cereals, dark green vegetables, Pulses, dried fruit, Parsley
Zinc	This mineral is also an antioxidant, and helps maintain a healthy skin and metabolism. It plays an important role in supporting the body's defence system and helps in the absorption of B vitamins	Seafood, Meat, Eggs, Wholegrain Cereals, Dairy Products, green vegetables, Pumpkin Seeds, Mustard
Iodine	Needed for the manufacture of key thyroid hormones which determine the rate at which our bodies work	Cows Milk, Seafood, Iodised Salt, Kelp
Selenium	A natural antioxidant that delays the oxidation of polyunsaturated fatty acids and preserves the elasticity of body tissue.	Wheat germ, Tuna, Tomatoes, Bran, Onion, Broccoli

	It helps to promote healthy blood flow and improves the function of energy producing cells. Also provides support for the immune system.	

Energy improving supplements

In addition to maintaining levels of all the above vitamins and minerals there are certain other supplements that are antioxidants and good at improving energy levels. Below is a selection of the ones I found most beneficial.

Alpha lipoic acid

This is both water and fat soluble and is a powerful antioxidant that enhances the activity of Vitamins C and E. It is manufactured in the body but not in the amounts that a tired body needs.

It supports the nervous system and is a key component of the metabolic process and produces energy in muscles and directs calories into energy production.

NAC N-Acetyl-l-Cysteine

Again this is a powerful free radical scavenger and supports the body's natural defence system.

Beta carotene

One of the major dietary antioxidants offering the body optimal nutritional support. It is a wonderful free radical scavenger and a powerful antioxidant that supports the body's defence system. The body converts beta carotene into vitamin A as needed.

Reduced glutathione

Another key component of the antioxidant system. It protects the body from free radicals. Reduced Glutathione is involved in the repair of DNA and also enhances the antioxidant activity of vitamin C, the transport of amino acids and the detoxification of harmful compounds.

CoQ10

This provides support to all cells of the body and is especially supportive of tissues that require a great deal of energy such as the heart and the cells of the body's natural defence system.

Echinacea

Helps the body's natural defence system, warding off infections.

Enada NADH – One of these a day made a dramatic difference to my energy levels

NADH stands for nicotinamide adenine dinucleotide, it is a coenzyme, present in all living cells, that helps in energy extraction and is made from vitamin B2, (niacin.)

By Acting as a coenzyme, NADH has an important role in helping enzymes to function as they should, breaking down food into energy for example.

In people, NADH stimulates the production of ATP (adenosine triphosphate), a compound that regulates the release of energy stored in cells. The more NADH a cell has, the more chemical energy it produces.

Research has also shown that increased concentrations of NADH in the brain may boost the production of neurotransmitters which are the brain chemicals vital to sound mental function.

Acetyl-L-carnitine

I found this really useful in promoting energy levels and improving my memory and attention span. It is found naturally in the body but again not in sufficient quantities if you are run down or very stressed.

Fatty acids

There is a growing trend to eliminate dietary fat, and indeed my own plan restricts the use of fat. However, certain type of fat is actually vital to good health. Essential fatty acids such as gama linolenic acid (GLA) and omega 3 fatty acids support a wide range of physiological functions. They cannot be manufactured by the body and must come from food or supplements. Unfortunately modern food processing removes many of these essential oils from foods. I found the following supplements useful

Black currant seed oil

This contains gamma linolenic acid GLA and can aid the immune system and joint health.

EPA/DHA

This is an ultra-pure fish oil concentrate and it helps maintain the blood flow and joint health.

Remember, each person's body is different and needs different amounts of vitamin and mineral supplementation. All the products carry a manufacturers' recommended dose and this should be followed unless you are advised by your doctor that you can take a larger quantity or know your own body well enough to know that a larger dose will help you.

Initially I took large doses of supplements and then reduced these as my energy levels improved.

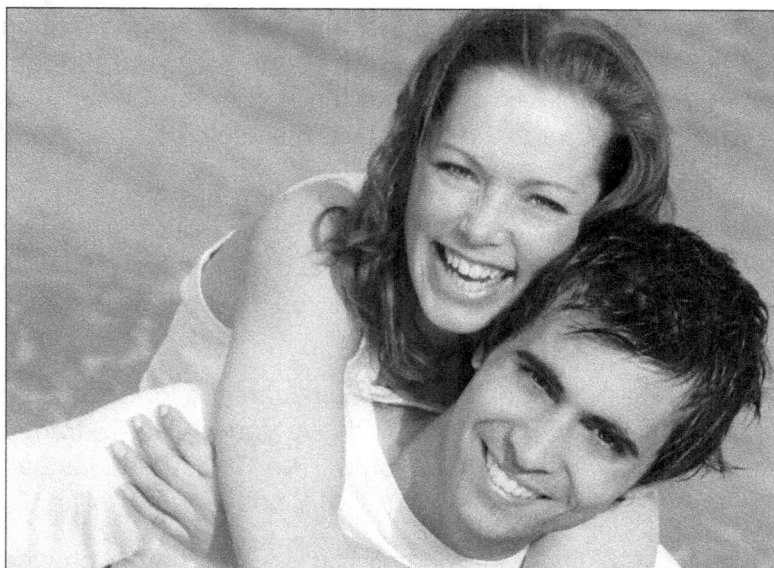

Conclusion
Ideas Worth Remembering

It's not the size of the dog in the fight that matters, it's the size of the fight in the dog.

You can and do create the life you want for yourself, the life that you think you deserve. You do it both consciously and sub consciously.

Take control of your negative thoughts and take control of your eating patterns and you can and will have a life filled with joy, happiness, enthusiasm, and excitement. You will have a life that rewards you for the effort that you have put in and a life that rewards others who are close to you as your "weather" rubs off on them.

Every system in your body is affected by your nutrition and every system in your body is affected by your thought patterns. The better your nutrition is and the better your thought patterns are, the better your self healing ability will be.

Eliminate your "what ifing...?", change your perception of every situation you face and live in the Now to fully experience all that life has to offer you. In other words, give your amygdala a rest.

Give your digestive tract a treat. Eliminate the foods that are causing toxins in your body and give your digestive tract a treat. Eliminate all the items on the No Go list, and instead fill yourself with the wide variety of foods on the Yes list.

Breathe new life into yourself, give your body a chance and give it a little exercise. Remember, Just 20 star jumps or jumping jacks each day can help eliminate toxic latent adrenalin.

You are in control, only you can change your situation. I urge you to make some changes and reap the benefits of a healthier, happier you.

Appendix

Oil and butter table

Family name	Members of the family
Cattle	Butter
Conifer	Juniper oil, Pine seed oil
Cotton	Cotton seed oil
Gourd	Pumpkin seed oil
Grass	Corn oil
Hazel	Hazelnut oil
Linseed	Linseed oil
Mustard	Rapeseed oil/margarine
Olive	Olive oil
Palm	Coconut oil/butter
Pea	Carob butter, Ground nut oil, Soya oil
Prunus rose	Almond oil, Apricot oil
Sesame	Sesame seed oil
Spurge	Castor oil
Sunflower	Safflower oil, Niger oil, Sunflower oil/ margarine
Walnut	Walnut oil

Flour and starch table

Family name	Members of the family
Banana	Banana, Arrowroot
Aroid	Dasheen arrowroot
Arrowroot	True arrowroot
Buckwheat	Buckwheat flower
Cyad	Sago, Florida arrowroot,
Ginger	Curcuma
Grass	Barley, Corn, Maize, Millet, Oat, Rice, Rye, Semolina, Wheat (do not eat wheat in first 3 months)
Palm	Coconut flour
Pea	Chick Pea, Green Pea, Gram, Lentil, Soya
Potato	Potato flour
Queensland	Queensland arrowroot
Sesame	Tahini
Spurge	Tapioca, Brazillian arrowroot
Sweet chestnut	Chesnut flour
Tacca	East Indian arrowroot, Hawaiian arrowroot

Herb table

Family name	Members of the family
Pepper	All types of peppercorns
Lily	Chive, Garlic, Sarsaparilla
Mint	Applemint, Basil, Bergamot, Bowles' Mint, Caraway, Thyme, Lavender, Lemon Balm, Lemon Thyme, Wild Thyme, Marjoram, Oregano, Rosemary, Sage, Summer Savoury, Winter Savoury
Grass	Lemon grass, Citronella
Ginger	Cardamom, Ginger, Turmeric
Sunflower	Tarragon, Tansy
Carrot	Angelica, Anise, Caraway, Chervil, Coriander, Cumin, Dill, Fennel, Lovage, Parley, Sweet Cicely
Avocado	Bay Leaf, Cassia, Cinnamon, Sassafras
Clove	Allspice, Clove
Iris	Saffron
Mace	Mace, Nutmeg
Orchid	Vanilla
Potato	Cayenne Pepper, Chilli, Paprika
Mustard	Horseradish, Mustard Seed
Citrus	Curry leaf
Buckwheat	Garden sorrel
Forget-me-not	Borage

Bibliography

Black C 17th March 2008 Working For a Healthier Tomorrow [Internet] Paper presented to Secretaries of Sate for Health and for Work and Pensions, Alan Johnson and James Purnell

Crowded House (1991) Woodface Album, Track, You Always Take the Weather With You (music)

Davidmann M How the Human Brain Developed and How the Human Mind Works [internet]

Griffiths L (2002) The Linden Method

Gschwandtner G March 2007 Great Thoughts to Sell By

Hill N (1937) Think and Grow Rich

MacLean P (1990) The Triune Brain in Evolution

Milton J Paradise Lost (1968) Longman Group Limited

Mohr B (1995) The Cosmic Ordering Service

Murphy J, MacMahn I (2000) The Power of Your Subconcious Mind

Tolle E (1997) The Power of Now: A Guide to Spiritual Enlightenment

Tolle E (April 2002) Practising the Power of Now

Twain M (2004) Mark Twain's Helpful Hints for Good Living: A Handbook for the Damned Human Race
"It's not the size of the dog in the fight that matters it's the size of the fight in the dog"